This
Is Your
Body on
Trauma

This Is Your Body on Trauma

How To Nourish Safety, Resilience, and Connection with Polyvagal-Informed Nutrition

Meg Bowman, MS, CNS, LDN, CHES

Health Communications, Inc.
Mt. Pleasant, South Carolina

www.hcibooks.com

Library of Congress Cataloging-in-Publication Data
is available through the Library of Congress

©2025 Meg Bowman

ISBN-13: 978-07573-2546-5 (Paperback)
ISBN-10: 07573-2546-7 (Paperback)
ISBN-13: 978-07573-2547-2 (ePub)
ISBN-10: 07573-2547-5 (ePub)

Publisher: Health Communications, Inc.
            1240 Winnowing Way, Suite 102
            Mt. Pleasant, SC 29466

Cover, interior design, and formatting by Larissa Hise Henoch

Contents

Supporting Safety from the Inside: A New Approach to Trauma and Nutrition

If you don't feel your feelings,
you get issues in your (body) tissues.

—Unknown

Erika arrived at the emergency room with a severe asthma attack less than an hour after finishing an appointment with her therapist. Just one month earlier, Erika, a thirty-two-year-old woman, had learned from a cousin that she had been sexually abused by a family member when she was very young—a truth her parents had known about at the time but had chosen to bury rather than address. In the weeks since the disclosure, her parents had been encouraging her to "forgive and forget" to keep the peace. Understandably, Erika was filled with rage at the parents who hadn't protected her then and still weren't protecting her now.

At home, Erika was having trouble sleeping, barely getting through the days with her newborn son. Every unexpected cry would send her into a startle response; she felt tense and constantly on edge.

After the abuse was discovered, during her therapy appointments, Erika felt so activated she could barely talk, and she told her therapist about often feeling tightness in her chest. But the therapist never would have guessed that just minutes after leaving her latest appointment, Erika would end up in the emergency room with an asthma attack.

Research helps explain why Erika's body reacted this way. After the September 11 attacks, studies showed that people who developed post-traumatic stress disorder (PTSD) were significantly more likely to experience severe asthma symptoms and to require urgent medical care. In fact, people with both asthma and PTSD were more than six times as likely to visit the emergency room with asthma compared to those who had asthma but did not develop PTSD.[1] It wasn't anxiety or depression that predicted these acute flares—it was the overwhelming body burden of traumatic stress itself.

Erika's story reflects this connection. Her nervous system, already shaped by early trauma, was now pushed into a survival state. Every unexpected noise, every confrontation with family, kept her system simmering at a near boil. The tightness in her chest, her restless sleep, her constant startle response—all of it pointed to a nervous system struggling to cope. The acute asthma attack wasn't separate from her trauma story; it was part of it.

I first heard Erika's story in a case consultation group, where a small circle of therapists—and me, a nutritionist—had gathered to discuss complex cases and support one another to find ways to better care for clients navigating trauma. Erika's therapist brought her case to the discussion, looking for support with her next steps. Should she help Erika dig deeper and process the trauma now, or should she tread lightly, protecting the fragile sense of safety Erika was trying to hold on to? The wound was so fresh, and Erika didn't seem ready—or able—to put her experiences into language yet. So what now? How do you support someone who can't talk about it?

There was a long pause. Eventually, I screwed up my courage and offered a suggestion. What if we didn't ask Erika to talk about the trauma just yet? What if we started with the body itself—supporting the physiological stress response that was fueling her asthma, her sleeplessness, her constant sense of threat—without requiring her to dive back into the painful memories? I suggested we try a bottom-up approach: nutrition.

By helping lower Erika's inflammation and nourishing her body with foods that supported her nervous system, we could start creating a foundation for physical safety. The goal wasn't to erase the trauma; it was to help her nervous system feel a little less under siege, even while her mind was still sorting through what had happened.

In my experience, this kind of bottom-up support can make a real difference. One therapist I often collaborate with once told me that having clients work with me makes her job at least 10 percent easier. She noticed that the clients with nutrition support seemed to have a stronger footing in therapy. They were better able to stay present during sessions, tolerate the discomfort that naturally arises when talking about trauma, and go deeper into their healing work. It wasn't that nutrition took away the pain. Instead, by calming the nervous system's internal alarm systems, it gave people just enough extra capacity to hold the hard things without becoming overwhelmed.

But while nutrition can be an incredibly powerful tool to support trauma healing, it's important to acknowledge that it can also be used in ways that cause real harm—especially when it's shaped by diet culture rather than by trauma-informed care. Unless we're really careful, the very tool that could help someone's ability to regulate and stay calm can instead become another source of rigidity, fear, and trauma. In the past decade, I've often seen how well-meaning providers, steeped in diet-culture thinking, have prescribed restrictive food rules without realizing they were retraumatizing their patients' already overwhelmed nervous systems. Instead of creating safety, these recommendations often deepened fear, shame, and disconnection—the opposite of healing. Here are just a few real examples of things my clients were told:

- "If you eat a cupcake for your birthday, even just once a year, you'll never get healthy"—said to a client dealing with inflammatory bowel disease. She had an excellent diet, normal labs, and her disease was currently in remission, but this proclamation caused her to question every single bite of food she put in her mouth for the next five years.
- "You should go on the carnivore diet. That's the only way to fix your mental health"—recommended to a client who had been a lifelong vegetarian for ethical and religious reasons.
- "You should go on an anti-candida diet to fix your ADHD"— recommended to a sixteen-year-old girl struggling with focus

at school. Six months later, she appeared in my office with anorexia, scared to eat anything after the anti-candida diet fueled beliefs that most food is "bad."

- "You should go on a five-day water fast to fix your diabetes"— the unhelpful recommendation given to a woman who had a ton of childhood food insecurity and was still wildly traumatized by even the thought of missing a single meal.

If we want to make nutrition a tool for healing, not harm, we have to rethink the approach entirely.

As sciences go, Western nutrition is pretty darn new. We're only about a hundred years into studying how food impacts health, and we're still figuring it all out. Many things I was taught in school ten years ago have since been proven incorrect. Some of the "absolute truths" presented at a conference I recently attended will likely be debunked in the next decade.

So how do we figure out what we *should* eat? In this book, I'm going to propose a new way forward that respects your nervous system's wisdom and honors the food survival strategies you've used to get here. Instead of tracking servings or counting macros, you'll learn to work with your body's trauma responses through food— using nourishment not as a set of rigid rules but as a tool to help you heal.

Let's get started.

A note to the reader:

In this book, I've deliberately simplified and consolidated information wherever possible, and I've chosen to write in a conversational style rather than academic or clinical language. There's a lot of complexity in the science behind trauma, the nervous system, and healing, but the last thing you need when you're dealing with the aftereffects of trauma is to feel overwhelmed or shut down by too much detail.

My goal is to give you enough understanding to make meaningful connections without drowning you in technical jargon or biochemical pathways. If you're interested and have the capacity to explore more, you'll find additional details and resources tucked into the sidebars throughout the book. You can dip into them if and when you feel ready—and you also have my full permission to skip them if that feels best.

Throughout the book, the stories and examples shared are composites, drawn from the experiences of many clients over the years. Names, details, and identifying features have been changed to protect privacy. While they reflect common themes I've seen in practice, they are not based on any single individual.

PART I
A Different Approach to Nutrition

If you picked up this book expecting a straightforward list of foods to eat and avoid, you might be surprised. Nutrition books often open with strict guidelines—cut this, add that, follow these rules, and you'll be healthier. But if you've ever tried to overhaul your diet only to find yourself overwhelmed, exhausted, or stuck in cycles of guilt and restriction, you already know that food is about more than just nutrients. The reality is that no set of nutrition rules will stick if they don't align with your nervous system's sense of safety.

That's why this book takes a different approach. Instead of starting with what's on your plate, we're going to start with what's happening inside your body after trauma—specifically, your nervous system. Your ability to make changes, maintain habits, and even recognize what foods feel good in your body depends on how regulated, safe, and supported you are. When stress, trauma, or survival mode take over, eating well can feel impossible—not because you don't know what to do but because your body is wired for protection, not optimization.

The first section of this book explores why food choices feel so complicated and why, despite our best intentions, it can be so hard to consistently eat in a way that supports health.

Chapter 1: Why Did I Get Sick?

This chapter reframes illness through a trauma-informed lens. Instead of blaming personal choices, we explore how chronic stress and unprocessed trauma disrupt the nervous system, leading to real physical symptoms like fatigue, digestive issues, inflammation, and autoimmune conditions. You'll learn how regulation, not restriction, is the first step toward healing.

Chapter 2: Why Is It So Hard to Eat Healthy?

If you've ever struggled to follow nutrition advice you know would help, you're not alone—and you're not lazy. This chapter explains how different nervous system states—like sympathetic activation or dorsal shutdown—impact appetite, energy, and motivation. It also explores how trauma drives both hypercontrol and disconnection around food and why adaptive, flexible eating starts with nervous system safety, not shame.

Chapter 3: Where Did My Relationship with Food Go Wrong?

Food is deeply tied to attachment, approval, and belonging. This chapter explores how early messages from caregivers, culture, or trauma shaped your eating patterns—whether through restriction, emotional eating, or complete disconnection. You'll learn how to identify the survival strategies behind your food behaviors and begin rebuilding trust with your body through safety and small, doable shifts.

Chapter 4: How Do I Choose a Way of Eating That Actually Works?

There is no one-size-fits-all diet—and following food rules that trigger stress or isolation can backfire, even if they're "healthy" on paper. This chapter helps you assess how your body responds to different nutrition approaches, avoid diet trends that aren't evidence based, and choose strategies that are not only effective but sustainable, affordable, and supportive of both health and connection.

For anyone who has ever felt like nutrition advice wasn't built for their reality, this book offers a different way forward. Rather than another set of rigid rules, this approach meets individuals where they are, honors the nervous system, and supports choices that are not just about food but about well-being, resilience, and lasting health.

CHAPTER 1

Why Did I Get Sick?

This isn't the Trauma Olympics.
You don't need to get a gold medal in
trauma to have experienced harm.

–Lotty Ackerman Mayer, LCSW

Tough times rarely arrive one at a time. Just when you think you've hit your limit, another challenge appears. This definitely was on my mind when I met Jen.

Jen was thirty-five when she was diagnosed with thyroid cancer. Thankfully, it had been caught early, and treatment only required surgery—no chemotherapy. Still, the experience shook her deeply. She had always considered herself healthy, and the diagnosis felt like it came out of nowhere. Even after a successful surgery, anxiety gripped her, disrupting her sleep, appetite, and sense of stability.

When we first met the week after her surgery, Jen complained of nausea and a frequent upset stomach. At first, I didn't find this surprising—it's pretty common to have post-surgery gut symptoms due to anesthesia and drugs used for pain management. But instead of resolving quickly, Jen's symptoms over the next few weeks grew to include frequent cramping and diarrhea nearly every time she ate.

Jen was so confused by her symptoms. "My gut has always been rock-solid," she told me. "Aside from some stomachaches when I was a kid, I've never had any issues. So why would this just start now?" Unfortunately, her symptoms weren't just limited to her gut. Jen became hypervigilant of *any* new sensation in her body. Even symptoms that had obvious causes sent Jen into a tailspin. The headache that was likely due to dehydration and resolved with an extra glass of water? That might be a stroke. The pain in her lower back likely caused by her weekend gardening? The cancer must have returned. Even though she objectively knew that she was safe, she didn't *feel* safe.

Because of her ongoing gut symptoms that still hadn't resolved after a month, at my prompting she went to a gastroenterologist who ran blood labs and performed a colonoscopy and endoscopy before diagnosing her with irritable bowel syndrome with diarrhea (IBS-D). The gastroenterologist's first recommendation was to try out some lifestyle interventions, like reducing Jen's intake of caffeine and alcohol and avoiding trigger foods. He also suggested she speak to me about a short-term low-FODMAP diet to assess for food triggers.

FODMAPs—short for fermentable oligosaccharides, disaccharides, monosaccharides, and polyols—are types of sugars found in certain foods that can be difficult for some people to digest, leading to bloating, gas, and diarrhea.[1] By temporarily removing high-FODMAP foods like onions, garlic, wheat, dairy, and certain fruits from Jen's diet, and then slowly reintroducing foods, the gastroenterologist hoped that Jen could identify which foods were contributing to her symptoms.[2] Over the next three months, Jen and I worked to implement the low-FODMAP diet, eventually identifying that her symptoms were primarily due to fructans, a type of oligosaccharide found in wheat, garlic, onions, bananas, and apples. When she ate less of those foods, the cramping and diarrhea improved significantly. While uncovering one of the food triggers for her gut symptoms brought Jen some relief—and slightly eased her anxiety—life continued to throw new challenges her way.

At a routine physical a few months after her IBS-D diagnosis, Jen's primary care doctor noted that her blood glucose was nearing prediabetes levels, and for the first time in her life she had high cholesterol and triglycerides. For Jen, it felt like her body was betraying her again. She had done everything right—followed medical advice, adjusted her diet, and taken care of her body—yet her health still seemed to be unraveling in ways she couldn't predict or control. It was frustrating, exhausting, and, most of all, deeply unsettling.

For Jen, the mounting health concerns weren't just physical. They triggered a familiar sense of instability, one that reached far beyond her recent diagnoses. Growing up in a home shaped by her mother's alcohol-fueled outbursts, she'd learned to stay hypervigilant, always scanning for danger, always preparing for the next blow—both figuratively and literally. Now, with her body throwing out new warning signals at every turn, it was like that same survival mode had been switched back on.

As we worked together, I started to wonder: Was Jen's body just reacting to the stress of her cancer diagnosis and surgery? Or was something deeper going on—something rooted in her past? Her nervous system had spent years in a state of high alert because of her childhood experiences. Could that old pattern still be running the show, contributing to the new health problems she was now facing? The more I listened to her story, the more obvious it became: This wasn't *just* about her thyroid, her gut, or her blood sugar. It was also about the wear and tear on her nervous system—and how old trauma was still shaping the way her body responded to triggers.

People like Jen remind me of a duck swimming across a pond. On the surface, to our friends and family, it looks like we're gliding through life, smoothly evading obstacles and moving toward our goals. But under the surface, our little webbed feet are paddling as fast as possible, just trying to stay ahead of the current. It reminds me of something Viola Davis wrote in her memoir, *Finding Me*, reflecting on the long shadow of childhood trauma: "And though I was many years and many miles away from Central Falls, Rhode Island, I had never stopped running. My feet just stopped moving."

Jen's story isn't unique. I've seen it time and again—people whose bodies seem to be fighting an invisible battle. The symptoms might shift and the diagnoses may differ, but the pattern stays the same: When stress, illness, or life throws things off course, it often stirs up old, unresolved trauma that shows up in the body.

Healing Requires More Than Willpower

Where Jen's experience is unique is the access she had to medical care. Her insurance allowed her to see specialists to support her conditions, see a therapist, and work with me at the same time. She had the time, energy, and cash on hand to implement the ideas we discussed.

This isn't the case for everyone. Health is not just a product of personal choices or willpower; it's also shaped by systemic forces such as racism, poverty, food insecurity, and by what happened to our ancestors. Healing requires more than just following medical or nutrition advice; it requires support, safety, and trust—things not everyone has equal access to. Unfortunately, access to safe, trauma-informed care is still a privilege, not a given.

So what was going on?

We often think of illness as something that happens to us—a virus, bad luck, genetics. But what if illness is also the result of how our nervous system has learned to respond to the world? When our bodies get stuck in chronic survival mode, they can no longer prioritize digestion, keep us from getting sick, or help us heal, which leads to chronic disease over time.

If you're like most clients I see who have experienced trauma, you've likely already been to talk therapy (I'm a big fan!), learned coping tools and techniques, listened to podcasts, processed your feelings, and more. And yet, you *still* don't feel at home in your body. Your nervous system continues to sense danger even though in most cases the danger has passed. Anxiety, depression, and focus issues are constant companions.

Something just *isn't right*. You've probably had the experience of being told by a physician that "everything's normal" when you know it's not. You seem to be racking up physical symptom after symptom and maybe have an autoimmune disease (or two). You're feeling either exhausted from trying therapy, diet, exercise, or random social media quick fixes or so shut down that trying anything feels impossible.

How do I know this? Like you, I've experienced trauma. Though I've done a lot of work to process my experience, I know what it feels like to have my body still "keep the score."[3] I've worked with countless clients who have had similar experiences. They experienced trauma, processed it to the extent they were able, and months or years later are chugging along with daily life, doing generally fine, when something happens to knock them right back into that traumatic state. They get headaches, gut problems, or crippling exhaustion. Sometimes it goes beyond temporary symptoms to medical diagnoses, such as IBS, autoimmune diseases, or diabetes.

But underneath the surface, the root causes for how we feel are rooted in something even deeper: how your nervous system continues to respond to the trauma you experienced. Without addressing the original root cause of trauma by finding safety in your nervous system, you'll get nowhere, and the next stiff breeze will knock you right back to square one. Chronic stress from trauma causes dysregulation in not only the nervous system but many of the body's other systems as well. This is how our lived experiences become our biology.

Finding Growth After Trauma

When we talk about trauma, we often focus on the harm it causes—and that's important. But there's another part of the story that doesn't get as much attention: post-traumatic growth.

Post-traumatic growth refers to the positive changes that can happen after we move through a traumatic experience. It doesn't mean that trauma is good or that we should be grateful for our suffering. It simply acknowledges that, alongside the real pain, people can sometimes discover unexpected strengths: a deeper appreciation for life, stronger relationships, new priorities, greater inner resilience, or a renewed sense of purpose.

Growth isn't automatic, and it doesn't erase the hurt. Healing takes time, safety, and support—and even then, growth looks different for everyone. Some people notice it quietly, like a new layer of patience or empathy. For others, it shows up as big life changes, such as changing careers, starting a creative project, or speaking up in ways they couldn't before.

You don't have to find the silver lining in your trauma. You're not failing if you're still in the messy middle. Post-traumatic growth isn't about pretending everything happens for a reason. Instead, it honors the ways in which it may be possible for you to grow through it.

Imagine an iceberg. The 10 percent you see above the water represents the physical and mental health symptoms you experience daily—fatigue, anxiety, pain, depression, or digestive issues. But beneath the surface lies the other 90 percent: the vast, hidden trauma guiding your nervous system's response that drives those symptoms upward, pushing them past the waterline, where they become visible. Without addressing this core issue—by creating a sense of safety and regulation in the nervous system—you're stuck. True healing starts not just by chipping away at the visible symptoms above the waterline but by addressing the submerged trauma that keeps them afloat.

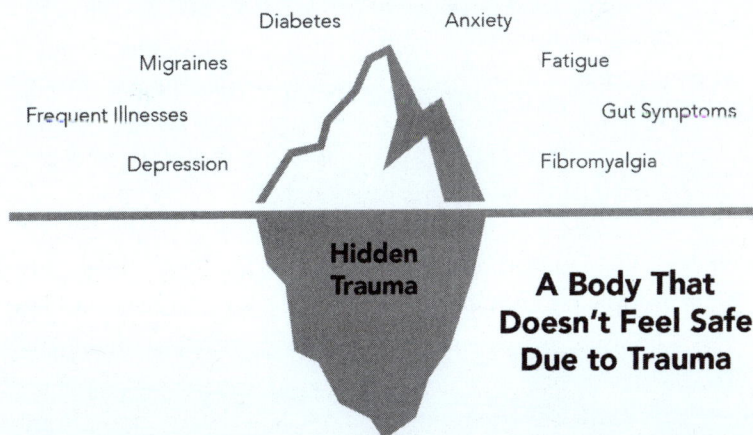

Diabetes   Anxiety
Migraines   Fatigue
Frequent Illnesses   Gut Symptoms
Depression   Fibromyalgia

Hidden Trauma

A Body That Doesn't Feel Safe Due to Trauma

Trauma can live beneath the surface, shaping symptoms that seem unrelated. What looks like fatigue, gut issues, or depression may actually be your nervous system responding to trauma.

Many of my clients are confused by their physical symptoms because they haven't experienced life-altering trauma such as Jen's—what we often call a "big T trauma." They believe that their daily, chronic experiences ("little t traumas") *shouldn't* have the same impact as a more acutely devastating event. But as Lotty Ackerman Mayer, the therapist of one of my clients, brilliantly noted, *"This isn't the Trauma Olympics. You don't need to get a gold medal in trauma to have experienced harm."* Our nervous systems tell our bodies to respond to threats in the same way, no matter whether that threat is a saber-toothed tiger or a nasty comment your aunt made at Thanksgiving.

Trauma Isn't Just One Thing

There are many different types of trauma that can impact both mind and body, some that will seem familiar and some that may not.

- Adverse childhood experiences (ACEs) are traumatic experiences that occur before we reach age eighteen. These include physical, emotional, and sexual abuse, as well as domestic violence, substance use or mental illness in the home, and incarceration of a family member. With each additional ACE we experience, our risk for disease goes up.
- Developmental trauma happens when our earliest experiences include inconsistent caregiving, emotional neglect, or environments that don't feel safe. This type of trauma often shapes our nervous system response to the world before we even have words for what we're feeling. I'm choosing to mention this separately from ACEs because developmental trauma isn't always captured by the ACEs framework—but it can have just as profound an impact on how we relate to ourselves, others, and the world.

- Chronic and complex trauma results from ongoing exposure to difficult experiences such as domestic violence, toxic relationships, bullying, systemic oppression, or being unhoused. To survive, the nervous system stays on alert for long periods of time without relief.
- Acute trauma includes one-time events such as a car accident, natural disaster, or sudden loss. Although the traumatic incident was time limited, the nervous system may continue to react to it long after it's over.
- Secondary trauma is common in people who help others through trauma. Healthcare workers, therapists, and first responders can be deeply affected by watching other people in pain.
- Collective, historical, and generational trauma doesn't just live in the past—it can echo through families, communities, and even the body. Some of this trauma is ongoing. For many, it's not just history; it's the present reality of living through war, systemic oppression, displacement, or the quiet, chronic stress of navigating life in a diaspora where parts of one's identity may feel unsafe or unwelcome. Research in the field of epigenetics shows that experiencing profound stress or trauma—especially during pregnancy—can alter the body's stress-response systems in future generations. These inherited changes don't necessarily come with memories or stories, but they can show up as heightened emotional sensitivity, a more easily triggered nervous system, or difficulty feeling safe or grounded.[4]
- Burnout can also cause trauma. While we often think of burnout as just being overworked or exhausted, severe or prolonged burnout—especially in caregiving roles

or high-stress environments—can create trauma-like
responses in the body.

Trauma makes it more likely that you will develop a disease, and it's not picky—it can affect every system in the body. People who have experienced trauma are more likely to have physical diseases such as asthma, high blood pressure, diabetes, fibromyalgia (FM), and IBS, as well as mental health conditions including addiction, anxiety, and depression. How does trauma create disease? It prevents your nervous system from feeling safe by keeping your body stuck in a survival state that prioritizes survival over repair.

Response to Threat: A Three-Act Play

Every human being has a basic biological need to feel safe. Our nervous systems are built to do exactly that: to scan for danger, take quick action to protect us, and then return us to a state of balance once the threat has passed. This automatic response isn't a flaw—it's a survival system, designed to keep us alive.

You've probably heard the well-worn story of the Neanderthal who crosses paths with a saber-toothed tiger. His sympathetic nervous system, part of our larger autonomic nervous system (ANS), kicks in, flooding his body with adrenaline that enables him to run away or fight off the tiger. If he can't get away or fight, his nervous system will induce a shutdown response so he appears dead and less interesting to the tiger. Then, once the danger is over, the Neanderthal returns to his normal routine of foraging for food. It turns out, in all these years, not much has changed with the human species! Our bodies are still wired to react with the same basic pattern of nervous system responses when we encounter a potential threat, which the work of scientist Stephen Porges helps us understand through polyvagal theory.[5]

The Roots of Resilience

Long before Stephen Porges conceptualized and described polyvagal theory, communities across the globe practiced regulation through song, movement, storytelling, breathwork, and connection with nature—approaches to regulation and resilience that you'll now see described on social media as "nervous system hacks."

Before polyvagal theory, we understood the autonomic nervous system as a seesaw. You either experienced sympathetic fight-or-flight energy *or* parasympathetic rest-and-digest energy. While one system was on, the other was off. In this model, it was expected that if you were stressed or activated, you could simply flip the switch—that regulation was something you could control with enough willpower.

An outdated view of regulation: on (sympathetic) or off (parasympathetic)

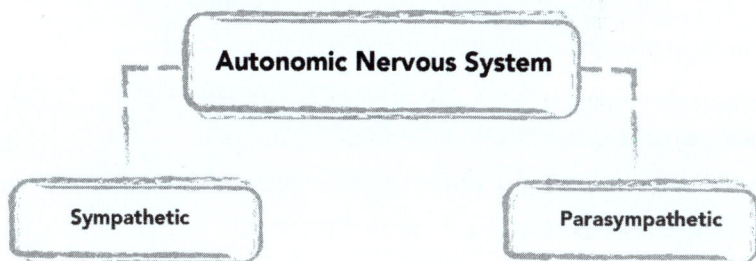

Autonomic Nervous System

Sympathetic

Parasympathetic

The traditional model of the autonomic nervous system saw it as a simple toggle switch—either fight-or-flight (sympathetic) or rest-and-digest (parasympathetic)—with no overlap or nuance.

I still see remnants of this way of thinking today. Stress was, and often still is, treated as a personal failure—if you can't calm down or relax, it means you lack discipline, strength, or character. Regulation was framed as a purely mental task: If you can "just think positive," "choose calm," or "just relax," everything will fall into place. For people who have experienced trauma, this misunderstanding can be especially damaging.

Today, endless social media memes encourage us to "self-care" our way out of distress—take a bubble bath, light a candle, go for a walk. While these suggestions may offer comfort for a nervous system that already feels safe, they often feel frustrating, hollow, or even shaming for someone whose system is stuck in survival mode. When the underlying trauma isn't addressed, surface-level self-care strategies rarely touch the deeper layers of dysregulation. For many trauma survivors, being told to "just relax" is not only ineffective; it reinforces the old belief that their struggles are a personal failing rather than a normal, adaptive response to an overwhelming situation.

Polyvagal theory gives us a new way to understand the nervous system, one that goes beyond willpower or mindset. It shows that our responses to stress aren't personal failures or character flaws; they're automatic, deeply wired survival strategies shaped by our past experiences. Instead of thinking of the nervous system as a simple "on-off" switch between fight or flight and rest and digest, polyvagal theory reveals a more layered map. It turns out that the parasympathetic system branches in two directions; one pathway (the ventral vagal) helps us feel safe and connected while the other (the dorsal vagal) can pull us into shutdown and collapse. In the next image, you'll see this updated map. Instead of telling someone to "just relax," polyvagal theory teaches us to meet the nervous system where it is and to gently support it to finding its way back to safety, connection, and resilience.

A polyvagal theory understanding of regulation: a continuum of nervous system responses

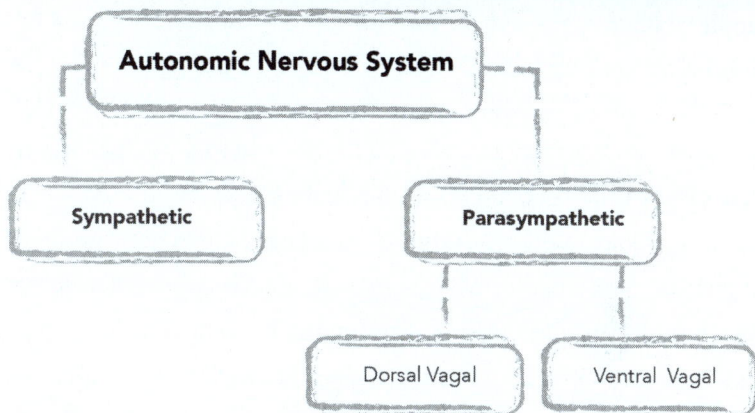

```
┌─────────────────────────────────┐
│   Autonomic Nervous System      │
└─────────────────────────────────┘
        │                 │
┌───────────────┐   ┌──────────────────┐
│  Sympathetic  │   │  Parasympathetic │
└───────────────┘   └──────────────────┘
                       │            │
              ┌──────────────┐ ┌──────────────┐
              │ Dorsal Vagal │ │ Ventral Vagal│
              └──────────────┘ └──────────────┘
```

Polyvagal theory expands our understanding of the nervous system beyond "on or off." Instead of a simple two-branch model, it recognizes three distinct pathways—sympathetic, dorsal vagal, and ventral vagal—each shaping how we respond to safety and threat.

If the old way of thinking about the nervous system was like flipping a light switch on or off, this new understanding is more like using a dimmer switch. There's a wide range of experiences between being in safety and survival mode.

When we talk about "vagal" responses in polyvagal theory, we're talking about how the vagus nerve helps shape the way we react to threats or to safety. The vagus nerve is one of the largest and most complex cranial nerves, connecting the brain to many key parts of the body, including the ears, throat, heart, lungs, stomach, and intestines. You can think of the vagus nerve as the main highway your survival messages travel on. Whether your body is sensing safety or danger, it's the vagus nerve that carries that information back and forth between your body and brain, guiding how you feel, think, and respond—often before you're even consciously aware of it. And when you're feeling relaxed and connected, it is also the vagus nerve that carries those messages of safety.

What's important to know is that most of the vagus nerve's work is bottom-up: About 80 percent of the nerve fibers are carrying information from the body to the brain, and only about 20 percent are sending information from the brain to the body. This means that most of the time, it's your body telling your brain how you're feeling—not the other way around. Your heart, lungs, gut, and other organs are constantly sending signals to your brain about whether the environment feels safe or threatening. In turn, your brain uses that information to shape your emotions, thoughts, behaviors, and even your sense of self.[6]

Deb Dana, LCSW (licensed clinical social worker), writes in her book *Polyvagal Practices* that the entire autonomic nervous system can be imagined as a ladder. At the top of the ladder is what she describes as the **ventral vagal** state, where we feel safe, healthy, and connected. As Dana describes it, "In this state our heart rate is regulated and our breath is full . . . we see the big picture and connect to the world and the people in it."[7] It's important to note that being in ventral doesn't mean you're always calm. You can cry, feel angry, be excited, grieve, or feel deeply emotional and still be in a ventral state. Regulated doesn't mean "happy" or even the absence of emotion, it means that you are connected and have the capacity to choose rather than react.

Polyvagal Ladder

Think of this ladder as a map of your nervous system.

The goal isn't to always be at the top—but to build awareness of where you are and how to climb back up when needed.

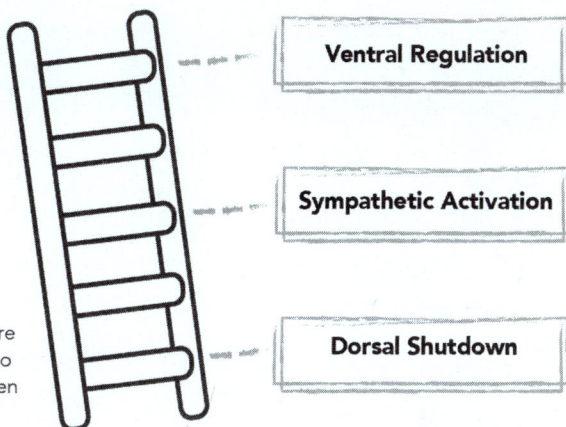

Ventral Regulation

Sympathetic Activation

Dorsal Shutdown

The Polyvagal Ladder
A visual metaphor for how we move through states of regulation and dysregulation, from connection (ventral) to activation (sympathetic) to shutdown and collapse (dorsal).

At the next level down the ladder, the **sympathetic** branch of the ANS activates when we feel uneasy, leading to fight or flight. Our heart rate speeds up, our breath is short, "we scan our environment looking for danger—we are on the move. . . . The world may feel dangerous, chaotic, and unfriendly. . . . Some of the daily living problems can be anxiety, panic attacks, anger, inability to focus or follow through, and distress in relationships."

At the bottom of the ladder is the **dorsal vagal** response, what Dana calls "the path of last resort. When all else fails, when we are trapped and action taking doesn't work, the dorsal vagal takes us into shutdown, collapse and dissociation."

A Note on Language

Throughout the rest of this book, I'll describe the body's survival states using the words *sympathetic activation* (for what polyvagal theory calls sympathetic) and *dorsal shutdown* (for

what's called dorsal). When I describe states of safety and connection, I'll use the words *ventral regulation*.

You might prefer different terms that feel more natural to
you. Some people use *hyperarousal* to describe sympathetic
activation and *hypoarousal* for dorsal shutdown. Others find
it helpful to think of these states simply as *too much energy*
or *too little energy*. There's no one "right" way to label your
experience.

As you read, I invite you to translate these words into whatever language you feel best reflects your nervous system's
experience.

In a perfect world, our nervous system would work like a well-
tuned alarm system: When something feels threatening, the alarm
sounds, our body responds, the situation gets resolved, and we return to feeling safe again. You can see this pattern clearly in babies.
When an infant feels scared, uncomfortable, or disconnected, she
cries or screams to show her distress. Ideally, a caregiver responds
quickly—soothing her, meeting her needs, and helping her nervous
system regulate. Over time, these moments teach her body that it's
safe to settle, and they help her build resilience to future stress.

And here's the key part: Once the danger passes and safety is re-
stored, the baby can go back to what she was doing—gurgling hap-
pily, playing with her toes, drinking her milk, taking in the world.
That full circle matters. True safety isn't just about avoiding danger;
it's about being able to return to connection and exploration afterward. We'll unpack why that's so important in just a moment.

We've evolved to complete certain actions in a certain order based
on our nervous system's cues. Like a chain of dominoes, certain
bodily functions and processes don't happen unless others happen
first. If the right cues don't trigger, we get stuck. But if we continue to

develop in a healthy way, then our tolerance for unexpected events or stressors grows with us, and we will be able to regulate our emotional and physical responses even when presented with new and novel situations.

Psychologist Abraham Maslow famously described human needs as a hierarchy, prioritizing our most fundamental needs for food, shelter, and physiological safety before the ability to create, explore, and grow.[8] And there's truth to this. Every teacher or parent who has ever tried to teach a hungry child knows that until the child gets fed, approximately zero critical thinking will occur. That child will put all their effort and energy into meeting that need for food and *not* into trying to learn advanced algebra. I have a seventeen-year-old son. Trust me, I know.

What's really important here is that until our safety needs are met, it's hard to make anything else happen. We get stuck. The domino stays standing. No passing go, no collecting $200. Our efforts at achieving those physiological needs—let alone the higher-order needs, such as deep relationships, education, career advancement, or pondering the lasting impact of the Roman empire—are thwarted until that sense of safety is restored. As therapist Deb Dana reminds us, "Story follows state," meaning that the lens through which we see the world is heavily informed by our nervous system.

Story Follows State
Your inner dialogue changes with your nervous system.

When you're in a survival state, it feels like . . .	• "People are against me." • "I have to keep pushing." • "There's no time to slow down." • "Nothing matters." • "I'm invisible." • "I can't do anything right now."
When you are regulated, it feels like . . .	• "I can handle this." • "I'm connected to the people around me." • "I trust myself to respond." • "I wonder what's possible." • "Mistakes are just part of learning." • "I can try new things safely."

Story follows state. What we believe, perceive, and expect from the world depends heavily on our nervous system state. The same situation can feel entirely different depending on whether we're in survival mode or in ventral regulation.

You can think of our body's response to threat—our attempt to find safety again—as following a three-part structure. As Bessel van der Kolk writes, it has "a beginning, a middle, and an end."[9] Just like a good play or story, there's a natural flow to how our nervous system reacts and recovers. And much like a play, it's not the work of one actor alone. It's a coordinated performance, with many parts of the body working together behind the scenes to keep us safe and bring us back to balance.

Act I: The Threat Appears

In June 1998, my college was hosting a summer music program for teens, and I was working there as a counselor. One night, there was a tornado warning as heavy thunderstorms swept across northeast Iowa, the wind pulling down hundreds of trees and launching flash floods in its wake. We gathered all the kids in a massive, windowless hallway inside the school cafeteria while the storm raged outside. One boy was experiencing an intense asthma attack and ran, unbeknownst to us, back to his dorm to get his inhaler. By the time he got back to the cafeteria, he was in major trouble. I had also suffered from asthma as a kid, so I recognized the severity of the situation due to his rapid breathing and coughing, as well as the way the skin at the base of his throat sucked in with each breath. Someone called an ambulance, and another counselor called his parents to alert them as well. While we waited for the ambulance to arrive, I stayed near him because I was the only counselor with any experience with asthma. Standing around waiting for the ambulance was awful. My heart was racing, I felt like my throat was closing up, and I couldn't stand still.

The moment that our earliest human ancestors came face-to-face with a saber-toothed tiger, the same automatic process began in their limbic brain, the earliest part of our brains to evolve. The limbic brain is home to the amygdala, which is responsible for registering threats and sounding the alarm. In terms of our three-act play, this is the inciting incident: the moment when ventral regulation is disrupted and we realize *all is not well*.[10]

Once the amygdala registers the presence of a threat, it sends a message to the hypothalamus along the hypothalamic-pituitary-adrenal (HPA) axis, setting off the world's fastest relay race. The hypothalamus releases a hormone that continues the journey along the HPA axis to the next stop, the pituitary glands, which in turn release adrenocorticotropic hormone (ACTH) to finally reach the adrenal glands. Message received, the adrenals flood the body with the stress hormones cortisol and adrenaline. Danger has been sighted, and the sympathetic nervous system leaps into action.

Cortisol's main job is to help us survive by putting nonessential body functions on hold. It raises our blood pressure, pulls sugar out of storage to give us a quick burst of energy, and sharpens our alertness so we can react fast. At the same time, it hits the brakes on systems we don't need in an emergency—such as digestion and immunity. After all, when you're facing a threat, it's not exactly the moment to focus on absorbing nutrients or fighting off a cold. Blood vessels tighten, energy gets rerouted, and the body shifts fully into survival mode.

While cortisol is busy shutting down the systems we don't need, adrenaline is flipping the switch on the ones we do. It redirects blood flow away from the digestive system and sends it toward the organs that will help us survive—such as the heart, which starts pounding, and the lungs, which open wide to gulp in more air. We get a surge of energy through our arms and legs, readying us to run, fight, cry, or scream if we need to.

Cue Act II.

Act II: Addressing the Threat

It took a long time for the ambulance to get to us. No wonder, really, given that they were trying to drive through tornado-level storms to reach us. In the meantime, other counselors gathered the campers away from me and the child with the asthma attack, and my mind raced. I tried to pull every ounce of data I'd ever heard about how to treat asthma out of my brain, but the only thing that came to me was a vague memory that caffeine helps with asthma. I sent another counselor along to the kitchen to make coffee while we waited, and eventually they came back with a mug, far too hot for anyone to actually drink.

When faced with danger, our nervous system empowers us to act. With adrenaline coursing through their veins, the ancient Neanderthal's nervous system had to judge whether they had enough time to flee from the saber-toothed tiger or they had to engage with it. This decision is made without conscious deliberation; our emergency response is so finely tuned that we can jump into action.

Interestingly, our response to threats changes when other people are around. As an evolved species, our nervous system has developed another first line of defense: social engagement. Instead of immediately jumping to a survival state, we first instinctively reach out—looking for connection, scanning faces, listening for voices that signal whether we're safe. As Stephen Porges explains, "In this hierarchy of adaptive responses, the newest social engagement circuit is used first; if that circuit fails to provide safety, the older circuits are recruited sequentially."[11] In other words, before launching into full-blown survival mode, your nervous system first tries to connect and coregulate.

When I first noticed the camper struggling, I instinctively glanced at the other counselors to see how they were reacting. Had they been calm, my nervous system might have stayed more grounded. But they looked panicked—and my own fight-or-flight response escalated in seconds.

But let's say that our nervous systems realize that fight or flight is impossible. What happens then? In the order of operations, we have a third defensive response available to us: we shut down. As Dr. James Gordon writes in his book *Transforming Trauma*, "When fight or flight and the stress response can't deal with an overwhelming and inescapable threat . . . a last-ditch survival mechanism, the collapse response, takes over." This response is monitored by the dorsal vagal complex, one of the oldest and most primitive parts of the brain, which only activates if it registers that escape is impossible. In that case, we enter a state of numbness and dorsal shutdown. Now, everything in the body slows as our nervous systems hope that by doing nothing, the danger will pass. Gordon writes, "When humans freeze, we may experience a self-protective detachment from our helpless, ravaged body, called dissociation."[12] While you may experience this state as a true immobilization, complete with difficulty moving, often people experience this state as a state of overwhelm, disconnection, or numbness.

Years later, I don't remember that ambulance ride at all, likely due to how traumatic it was for me. It all stemmed from my own childhood experience with asthma.

You see, I had a pretty crappy experience of asthma as a kid. Although my asthma symptoms wouldn't have been classified as severe, my experience of it was. The symptoms themselves were terrifying, like trying to gulp air through the world's smallest straw. And my anxiety didn't end when the asthma attack did. I know it's hard to imagine, with today's asthma prevalence rates, but at the time, I was the only kid in my grade (maybe even in my school) with asthma, which made me feel isolated. I had to avoid certain activities such as sleepovers with a friend whose parents smoked.

My parents did their part to try to relieve my anxiety, providing a ton of education and support, and even got me an asthma board game so I could better understand what was happening to me. But the whole asthma experience was still super scary, and I never knew when an attack would hit. Soon, the anxiety that came with an asthma attack became associated with other things. I started to avoid the area of the house where the asthma board game was stored, and I tried diligently never to look at the bookshelf (second from the bottom, on the left side) that it was on. I experienced a moment of anxiety walking into restaurants because in those days—when smoking was allowed in many indoor spaces, including airplanes—wafts of smoke would come over to the nonsmoking side from the smoking side. All of it triggered my asthma, and it felt like nowhere was safe. Luckily, by age twelve, I had grown out of asthma, but the anxiety that had become hardwired in my brain to go *with* asthma remained.

So when I saw that camper dealing with an asthma attack, my anxiety came roaring back—even though the camper's symptoms resolved quickly once we got to the hospital. I remember calling his parents later and asking whether they wanted to pick him up. He was safe and happy, so they were fine with him staying at camp. The storm had subsided.

For everyone but me.

You've likely experienced all these responses at different times in your life, depending on the context, environment, and severity of the danger. A survival state could be activated in any number of daily events where we might, consciously or subconsciously, feel threatened. These events don't have to be as dramatic as facing a saber-toothed tiger or riding in an ambulance through a tornado. You could experience any of these reactions even in the face of "smaller" dangers, such as receiving criticism from your boss, watching the news, or experiencing turbulence on an airplane. You don't consciously think about which response is appropriate; your nervous system filters through these options subconsciously to find the one most likely to keep you safe.

When this process happens successfully and we're able to avoid, escape, or neutralize the danger, we start Act III.

Act III: Safety Restored

After I went back to campus later that night, a bunch of counselors decided to go to a pizza restaurant to relax. I went along, thinking maybe that would help to calm my own nerves, too. But as I sat in the booth in the basement of the restaurant, unable to touch my food and desperate not to show others what was happening, the world felt like it was shrinking. I didn't know it, but I was in the midst of my first full-fledged panic attack. My throat was closing, my heart was pounding, and my stomach felt like it had dropped straight into the center of the earth itself. Something was very, very wrong.

Just hours after I had left the hospital with the camper, I went back to the emergency department. None of the doctors could identify anything wrong with me physically. It certainly wasn't an asthma attack; I knew what that felt like. One doctor suggested that I was probably having a reaction to the antibiotic I was on at the time, and I was sent home to recover. For decades after that, I believed that I was allergic to penicillin (I'm not).

The only thing "wrong" with me was that my nervous system wasn't able to get back to safety, back to a ventral state of regulation. But why not?

Let's say our ancestor manages to outrun the tiger. Once the danger passes, the amygdala sends out the all-clear signal: We're safe. That's the cue for the parasympathetic nervous system (PNS) to step in and take over. The stress response quiets down, cortisol and adrenaline levels drop, and the vagus nerve sends a new message through the body: It's time to return to homeostasis. Blood flow returns to the digestive tract, the immune system kicks back into gear, and the body shifts from defense mode to repair mode. Digestive enzymes are released, muscles relax, and the food moving through the gut can finally be broken down and absorbed—allowing the body to nourish and heal itself again.[13]

All is as it should be, *should* being the operative word.

I've drawn my experience below, showing the shift from connection and social engagement with the other counselors prior to the tornado (ventral regulation), through alarm and action (sympathetic activation) to dissociation (dorsal shutdown), and then back into the alarm stage (sympathetic activation) at the pizza restaurant. You'll notice that at no point during this incident did my nervous system get all the way back into connection and safety. In the months that followed, I spent a lot of time stuck in sympathetic activation—hyperaware of everything around me, with my body on constant alert every time I left the house.

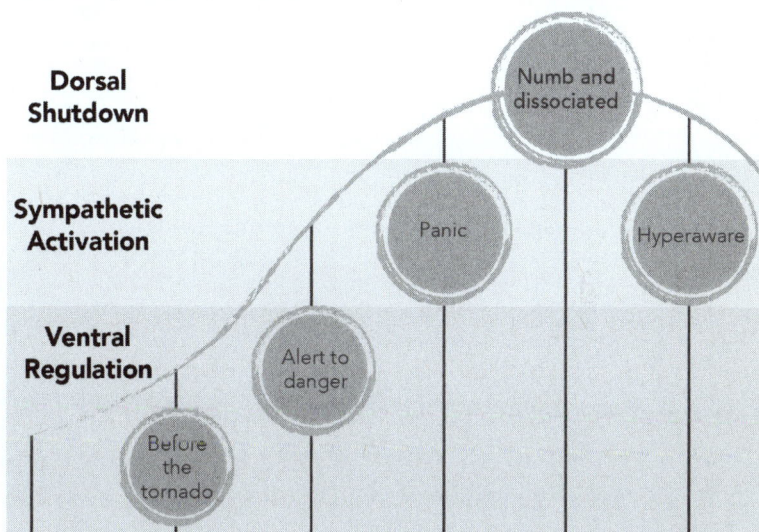

Dorsal Shutdown — Numb and dissociated

Sympathetic Activation — Panic — Hyperaware

Ventral Regulation — Alert to danger — Before the tornado

Your nervous system remembers what your brain might forget. When trauma loops through your nervous system, the path back to safety isn't always linear—but healing begins when we learn to map the way.

This image maps my nervous system's journey through trauma, following me from connection before the tornado (ventral regulation) into sympathetic activation (a panic attack) and then dorsal shutdown (dissociation). It also shows how I cycled back into activation without fully returning to safety, showing how trauma can disrupt the natural rhythm of regulation.

Panic attacks became a regular occurrence in my life, and I spent the rest of that summer terrified to leave the house in case one hit. Eventually, my triggers spread in a process that licensed social worker and trauma expert Linda Thai calls being "hashtagged together." Since my trauma involved tightness in the chest, I became hyperfixated on, and scared of, any cough or illness #colds #flu but also #coldair and #sickpeople. Swallowing food became scary too. If you've ever accidentally inhaled a little bit of food or liquid, you can imagine how similar this feels to asthma #choking #smallbites. Because this all happened in a basement, I started fearing #undergroundparkinggarages and #roomswithnowindows. And I definitely didn't want anyone to see me struggle, #hide. None of this was happening in my prefrontal cortex (i.e., my logical brain). It often wasn't even conscious. It just was what life felt like. My nervous system got stuck in "danger" mode, with no way to get out.

Our nervous systems are constantly scanning for signs of danger and safety, a process Stephen Porges calls "neuroception."[14] The problem is, we're wired to detect threats far more easily than we recognize safety—and in today's fast-paced, unpredictable world, those signals of danger are everywhere. It's not just the jolt of adrenaline when your car skids on the ice. It's the drip, drip, drip of bad news. You get an alert about another school shooting, hear about another looming pandemic on the news, and talk with your neighbors about the rash of unsolved burglaries in your neighborhood. All of it keeps our systems on edge and leaves us feeling like the world is coming apart.

Sometimes, the cues that trigger this survival response are incredibly subtle. I saw this firsthand with my client, Alice. One Tuesday morning, during our session, the tornado sirens in my town went off for their routine weekly test. For just a brief moment, my attention flickered as I instinctively checked whether it was an actual emergency or just the usual test. I quickly realized it was Tuesday at 10 AM—nothing to worry about—but Alice had already caught something in my face. She saw my microexpression—the split-second seriousness as I assessed for danger—and even without conscious thought, her nervous system filled in the gaps. To her, that flicker of concern on my face didn't register as me reacting to a siren; it brought her straight back to the way her mother's face would tighten in anger whenever she did something "wrong." In that instant, Alice wasn't just reacting to the sound outside—she was responding to an old, familiar fear of disapproval and rejection, a pattern shaped long ago by experiences she hadn't yet put into words.

That's neuroception in action. It runs in the background, outside of our awareness, scanning for subtle changes in our surroundings and in the people nearby. Maybe your heart speeds up, your breath shortens—and before you even realize it, your brain is already spinning a story to explain why.

Danger signals don't just come from outside our bodies; they can also come from inside, often without us even realizing it. Imagine someone who grew up with a parent who had explosive anger. As an adult, they might feel a sudden wave of discomfort during a work meeting, even though nothing obviously threatening is happening. Their heart rate speeds up, their breathing gets shallow, and their stomach tightens. They may not realize that a coworker's slightly raised voice or a flash of frustration on someone's face has triggered an old memory of danger. Even though their logical brain knows they're safe, their nervous system has already decided otherwise, shifting them into a survival state.

This can happen with physical sensations too. A racing heart from drinking coffee or feeling lightheaded from low blood sugar can be misread by the nervous system as a sign of immediate danger, sometimes even triggering anxiety or a panic attack. The body reacts first before the mind has a chance to catch up and make sense of it.

These nervous system "mismatches"—when you are objectively safe, but your body doesn't feel safe—are incredibly common after trauma.

Helping the Body Feel Safe Again

The brain and body can stay stuck in "high alert" mode—always watching for danger, even when we're safe. This constant state of stress makes it hard for the body to relax, heal, or function normally. That's why intentionally sending the body clear signals of safety is so important for healing. When the body feels safe, its systems—such as digestion, immunity, and hormone balance—can return to a state of rest and repair.

This brings us back to Jen, whom we met at the start of the chapter. Her story shows a reality we rarely acknowledge: Illness is often more than just a collection of symptoms or a diagnosis. It's a reflection of how our bodies have learned to survive. When we experience chronic stress or unresolved trauma, our nervous system gets stuck in a loop of hypervigilance, keeping our body in a constant state of defense. Over time, this wears down key systems: our digestion, immune function, metabolism, and even our ability to rest and recover.

If we only focus on treating symptoms—taking medication for gut issues, adjusting diet for blood sugar, or managing anxiety with talk therapy—we're addressing the surface of the problem without getting to the core of why our body is reacting this way in the first place. Until we help the nervous system recognize safety again, healing remains incomplete, and the body continues to send distress signals in the form of illness, inflammation, and exhaustion.

The good news is that this process isn't irreversible. Just as the nervous system learned to stay in survival mode as an adaptive protection response, it can also learn to shift back more frequently into a state of ventral regulation and healing.

But here's something important to understand: If you have a trauma history, change can feel especially hard. Trauma can teach us that familiar is safe—even if the familiar isn't healthy. New patterns, even ones meant to support healing, can feel risky or unsafe at first. That's not a failure. It's your nervous system doing exactly what it was trained to do: protect you. Real healing often means going slow.

So, if you've ever felt like Jen and you are wondering why your health is unraveling despite doing all the "right things," know that you're not broken or alone. Your body is responding exactly as it was designed to. The key isn't just managing symptoms; it's understanding the deeper nervous system messages your body is sending and finding a way to restore balance, one step at a time.

In the next chapter, we'll explore how the body's survival responses of sympathetic activation and shutdown, once used to protect you, may now be keeping you stuck, making it difficult to feel regulated and eat in a healthy way.

CHAPTER 2

Why Is It So Hard to Eat Healthy?

We didn't know who we would be.
We didn't know where we would end up
When we headed down that road.

—Antje Duvekot, *Long Way*

Every nutrition provider I know has a list of "divisive foods" that, when mentioned to a client, are either going to be a huge win or something to avoid at all costs. Read through the list below, tune into your body signals, and see how you react to the thought of eating these foods. Pay special attention to the foods that bring you joy or excitement, as well as the foods that bring a feeling of disgust or nausea.

41

Highly Divisive Foods

Foods that people tend to either love or hate, with little in between!

Anchovies	Green bell peppers	Sardines
Black licorice	Herring	Sea urchin (Uni)
Blue cheese	Kimchi	Sour cream
Brussels sprouts	Liver	Spam
Cilantro	Marmite/Vegemite	Sushi (especially
Coconut	Mayonnaise	raw fish varieties)
Cottage cheese	Mushrooms	Tempeh
Durian	Okra	Tofu
Eggplant	Olives	Truffle oil
Fennel	Oysters	Wasabi
Ginger	Papaya	
Goat cheese	Pickled eggs	

This list includes some of the most polarizing foods—ingredients people tend to love or loathe. Notice how your nervous system reacts to each one as you read through.

Did any foods on that list bring up a challenging reaction in your body? That's the feeling of extra stress on your system, and you likely just experienced mild sympathetic activation or dorsal shutdown energy. You likely aren't experiencing full-on panic attack (or maybe you are—cilantro really scares some people!), but it's possible that just the thought of the hated food changed your nervous system energy.

If you loved every single food on the list and didn't notice much change, that's great too! In that case, think about something that feels mildly uncomfortable or scary to you—such as holding a spider or giving a big speech—and tune into how your nervous system responds. Your body is always sending you signals; the goal here is simply to start noticing them.

Now, I'd like you to imagine that you read a study that said the only way for you to get healthy was to eat a food that you hate every single day.

How do you think that would play out?

Probably not well.

You might get frustrated with the advice, try to force yourself to follow it, feel ashamed when you couldn't, and eventually give up altogether—not because you lacked willpower but because forcing your nervous system into an extreme state of stress almost never leads to lasting change.

On paper, eating right looks easy—"Eat this many servings of these food groups, don't overdo sugar or salt, and you'll be fine." In reality, eating well can be incredibly difficult—especially for people who have experienced trauma and whose bodies spend a lot of time stuck in survival mode. When we're in a survival state, we don't have much conscious capacity for choice; our nervous system is too busy trying to keep us safe to prioritize thoughtful decision-making. Folks, it is really hard to read a menu when the building is on fire. Ventral regulation—the ability to feel connected and grounded—is what gives us the space to actually choose how we want to eat instead of reacting automatically to stress.

This is where the shift from the old way of thinking about the nervous system to the polyvagal-informed model makes a huge difference. In the old "seesaw" model, if you were stressed, the advice would be simple: Just calm down. Take a few deep breaths, muster some willpower, and make the "right" choice. In reality, if your nervous system is stuck in a state of sympathetic activation or dorsal shutdown, it's not a matter of willpower—it's biology.

Imagine a mom with three kids under the age of five just finished a full workday, raced through daycare pickup, and on the way home realized there was nothing in the fridge to make for dinner. She's completely exhausted, her nervous system on high alert from a day of multitasking and caregiving. On the way home, she swings through the drive-thru for fast food. In the old model, someone might say she made a "bad choice" that she should have resisted.

But from a polyvagal perspective, we recognize that her survival brain prioritized quick energy, minimal effort, and immediate relief; her system was operating from an activated place of perceived threat and exhaustion, not regulated long-term planning. Instead of blaming her for the choice, we would focus on helping her build more moments of safety and ventral regulation into her day so that next time, she actually has the internal capacity to choose.

Polyvagal theory reminds us that if we want different outcomes, we have to start with safety, not shame.

By this point it should be clear that when the nervous system perceives a threat—real or imagined—it shifts into a survival state to protect us. In that state, the way we respond can vary. Some people feel depleted and shut down. Others feel a sudden surge of energy and an urgent need to take action. Either way, trauma makes it even harder to regulate the nervous system enough to make thoughtful, balanced food choices.

If someone has a history of food insecurity, for example, even the idea of changing their diet can trigger fear and urgency. Scarcity feels dangerous to a nervous system that once went hungry. Someone who grew up with overly strict parents who controlled what or how much they ate might find that any attempt to "eat healthy" stirs up old feelings of deprivation or rebellion. Even traumas that aren't directly about food—such as medical trauma, childhood neglect, or sexual assault—can leave the nervous system in a chronic state of dysregulation, making consistent, nourishing eating feel impossible.

This is why eating well isn't just about willpower or nutrition knowledge. It's about whether your nervous system is in a place where you can actually access choice—where you can respond thoughtfully instead of automatically reacting from a place of survival.

Your body is incredibly good at helping you survive. When you're faced with trauma or high stress, it shifts your resources to focus on getting you through the danger. One of the ways it does this is by releasing a chemical called corticotropin-releasing hormone (CRH), which not only helps you respond to the threat but also suppresses your appetite.[1] In the short term, this is a smart survival move; if you're running from a tiger, stopping for a snack isn't exactly a priority. But when stress becomes chronic, that same appetite suppression can start to backfire, putting you at real risk for malnutrition and further depleting your body's reserves over time.[2]

Prolonged stress, on the other hand, can actually *increase* your appetite.[3] When stress sticks around, your body releases hormones called glucocorticoids, which tell the brain's hypothalamus to rev up hunger signals. These hormones make you produce more ghrelin (the hormone that makes you feel hungry) and make you less sensitive to leptin (the hormone that signals fullness). As a result, you not only feel more hungry, but it also takes more food to feel satisfied.[5] Prolonged stress also promotes insulin resistance, which can make cravings for high-fat, high-sugar comfort foods even stronger. And here's the thing: This isn't a failure of willpower—it's your body doing exactly what it's designed to do to survive. Studies show that eating "highly palatable" foods can actually help soothe stress in the short term.[4] That's why reaching for comfort food when you're under stress often feels automatic. Even if it's frustrating, this is your body's adaptive way of trying to protect you by making sure your brain has enough fuel to deal with hard things. Food brings comfort and a sense of relief when you need it most.

Why Your Body Reaches for Cookies, Not Kale, Under Stress

Reaching for foods high in sugar, fat, or salt during stress is a commonly used coping strategy. These comforting foods can help regulate the nervous system and bring a sense of relief or stability, even if just for a little while. But over time, relying on this strategy as your *only* option to regulate can become maladaptive by potentially contributing to inflammation and altering hunger and fullness cues.

When working with clients, I never know exactly how their nervous system will respond to stress—whether it will increase or suppress their appetite—but I almost always expect some impact. After the Russian invasion of Ukraine in 2022, researchers studied 619 refugees who had relocated to Germany, examining their eating behaviors in relation to psychological distress. They found that 58.5 percent experienced changes in appetite: 46.3 percent ate less while 12.2 percent ate more.[5]

Why do some people lose their appetite under stress while others turn to food for comfort? It's a mix of both biology and emotion. One study found that people with lower levels of ghrelin needed more high-fat, high-calorie foods to feel satisfied and shut off their stress-driven hunger.[6] Others, however, had the opposite reaction— their nervous system responded to danger by shutting down appetite altogether. How your body reacts to stress plays a powerful role in shaping your relationship with food—often more than willpower or good intentions.

When "Healthy Eating" Leaves People Out

A lot of what gets called "healthy eating" isn't neutral; it's shaped by culture, privilege, and power. Many mainstream nutrition guidelines reflect Western, white, middle-class values, while traditional and culturally important foods—such as rice, plantains, fermented dairy, or animal fats—are often left out or even labeled as "bad."

At the same time, there's huge emphasis placed on expensive foods such as organic produce, grass-fed meats, and time-consuming meal prep. When these become the gold standard for "health," food choices get moralized, and anyone who can't (or doesn't want to) follow them may be unfairly judged as irresponsible, lazy, or unhealthy. But health isn't one-size-fits-all. True nourishment honors culture, accessibility, and lived experience—not just a rigid set of rules.

In contrast to what diet culture–fueled social media posts would have you believe, the first step in eating healthy isn't choosing what to eat or not to eat, it is learning more about how your nervous system responds to stress.

Polyvagal therapist Deb Dana invites clients to discover their "home away from home," or default survival state.[7] While everyone will experience both sympathetic activation and dorsal shutdown from time to time, your "home away from home" is the survival state that feels more familiar to you, or that happens more often. As you read through the following client examples, pay attention to whether one state or the other feels more familiar.

Sympathetic Activation

Stress kicks some people into overdrive. Instead of feeling paralyzed, they respond to a crisis with urgency, hypervigilance, and an overwhelming need to act. These are the people who, when faced with a health scare, immediately research every possible treatment, overhaul their diet overnight, stack their supplement routine with precision, and double down on control in an attempt to outmaneuver uncertainty.

This was exactly how Jan, a fifty-three-year-old health coach, responded after her breast cancer diagnosis. While her drive to "fix" things initially felt empowering, it quickly spiraled into an exhausting, all-consuming mission—one that left her more anxious and depleted than before. Jan had recently finished treatment for breast cancer and was understandably still reeling with anxiety and experiencing regular nightmares. A year before I met her, when she was first diagnosed, she chose to go on a gluten-free, dairy-free, soy-free, grain-free, sugar-free, vegan diet that was much more restrictive than the plant-based diet recommended by her oncologist. Instituting hard-and-fast rules about food was the way she coped. But changing her food wasn't the only thing she did.

For Jan, managing her danger signals necessitated twice-daily saunas, installing a whole-house water filtration system, stopping eating out entirely, taking twenty-five different supplements (I'm not kidding; she brought them to our first session in a paper grocery bag), and seeing a chiropractor, massage therapist, acupuncturist, along with me, each week. Now, for all the haters out there who are going to be mad at me and say that she was doing all those things to get healthy, okay, sure. But trust me when I say that none of these things relieved her anxiety; in fact, they increased it.

I first met Jan six months prior to her son's wedding, when she made an urgent appointment with me because she was both terrified *to* take a bite of cake at the wedding in case it would make her cancer return and terrified *not* to eat the cake in case everyone around would realize just how restrictive her eating patterns had become.

The cancer diagnosis was the trauma, and the restrictive eating patterns were her coping response.

Her response indicated sympathetic activation, the drive to "fix it *now*" that I see so commonly in people who have experienced or are experiencing trauma. I'm not saying that activated energy is always problematic. It's not. You need some amount of sympathetic activation to be able to get up in the morning and go about your day. If you've ever played a sport or even just a rousing round of checkers, you've likely experienced sympathetic activation blended with ventral regulation. Jan used this blend of energy successfully when she got a second opinion from another oncologist and started to build a supportive team of providers. But sometimes, when left unchecked and without blending with ventral regulation, sympathetic activation energy can create hyperfixation and hyperawareness, building anxiety and preventing you from seeing other possibilities. While that move into an activated state was initially adaptive for her, staying there resulted in many decisions that were maladaptive over time. Jan got stuck in survival mode and couldn't get out.

In addition to the "fix-it" response, I've seen a number of different sympathetic activation responses in my clients while trying to focus on their health. Do any of these feel familiar to you?

Hyperfixation on the "Perfect" Health Plan

- Hyperfixation on finding the "perfect" diet or health regimen
- Constantly researching, seeking the "best" or "cleanest" way to eat
- Signing up for an expensive wellness program, detox, or protocol overnight without considering sustainability
- Seeking multiple second opinions or working with several practitioners at once on the exact same things

- Feeling impatient if symptoms don't improve immediately, and switching protocols frequently

Strict Control over Food and Exercise

- Relying on calorie counting, macro tracking, or fitness apps with rigid adherence
- Feeling distressed if you miss a day of tracking or don't meet self-imposed goals
- Taking an excessive number of supplements to feel "in control" of your health

Pushing the Body Beyond Its Limits

- Engaging in intense, high-impact workouts even when exhausted
- Finding it hard to engage in gentle movement such as yoga, walking, or stretching because it doesn't feel productive
- Feeling unable to rest or recover, fearing you will lose progress
- Feeling like rest is "wasting time"

I've found that people who default to sympathetic activation mode often *do more instead of feel more*. These people believe that if they just try harder, do more, or get everything "right," they'll finally feel better. But instead, their nervous system remains stuck in high alert, preventing true ventral regulation and healing.

Diet culture thrives on keeping us stuck in survival mode, pushing people to approach food with urgency, hypervigilance, and a constant need to "prove" their virtue through clean or disciplined eating. The endless pressure to count calories, track macros, cut out food groups, or stick to rigid meal plans keeps the nervous system in a state of stress. It teaches people that their food choices must be tightly controlled to be healthy, worthy, or good enough.

This is how sympathetic activation hijacks your plate.

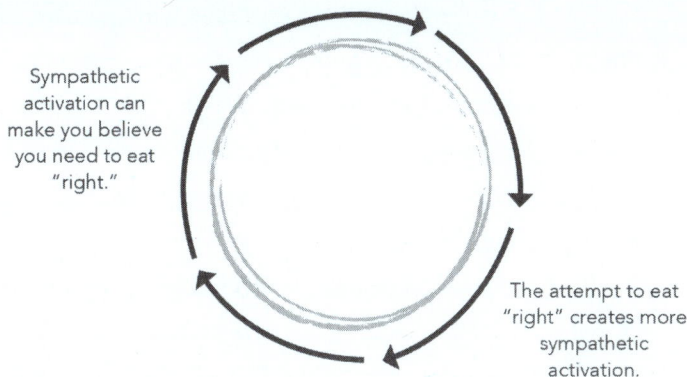

Sympathetic activation can make you believe you need to eat "right."

The attempt to eat "right" creates more sympathetic activation.

Even well-intended food rules can keep us stuck. Stress about eating "right" often leads to more stress—and further from the nourishment we truly need.

When you're stuck in this kind of sympathetic activation, it's easy to lose touch with your natural hunger and fullness cues. Instead of trusting your body's signals, you end up eating based on fear, external rules, or shame. This often leads to a familiar cycle: restrict certain foods, feel deprived, rebel against the restriction, then feel guilty after eating "bad" foods.

Over time, this disconnect from your body weakens your ability to recognize when you're actually hungry, satisfied, or in need of nourishment. Food becomes a source of stress instead of support, and the nervous system stays locked in the very survival patterns that make sustainable, balanced eating so difficult to find.

Dorsal Shutdown

If Jan's story doesn't resonate with you, I'm guessing you might lean more toward a state of overwhelm or dorsal shutdown. That was the case of Dani, a thirty-four-year-old mother of twin toddlers who came to me with complaints of chronic fatigue, lethargy, and chronic heartburn.

Dani reached out on the advice of her therapist but was the first to acknowledge her ambivalence. "I don't know why I'm here," she said during our first session. "I know I should take better care of myself and avoid the foods I know trigger my reflux, but I can't bring myself to do anything about it. I just don't have it in me." Dani had been struggling for years with GERD (gastroesophageal reflux disease), feeling persistent heartburn and pain after eating. She knew that coffee, fried foods, and chocolate triggered her symptoms, but even with that knowledge, she felt stuck. She told me that coffee was the only way she could drag herself out of bed in the morning. In fact, when asked about her food habits in the intake paperwork, Dani wrote "Don't take away my coffee!!!"

Dani's health history revealed a traumatic past. As a child, she lived in a house with parents who drank too much and had roaring fights when drunk, often to the point that neighbors would call the police. Dani spent many nights sitting in a closet in her room in the dark waiting for the fighting to end. "When the fighting started, I'd just go numb," she explained. "It was like my body wasn't mine anymore, and I'd just disappear into the darkness of the closet. I stayed as still as possible, barely breathing, until it was over."

That deep, protective dorsal shutdown response became a default pattern for Dani whenever she felt overwhelmed. As you can probably imagine, overwhelm happened regularly with two energetic and loud toddlers in the house. Like most parents of young kids, Dani felt exhausted most days, but her exhaustion went further than just feeling tired. She also felt disconnected from her body and needs and felt numb.

By the time she came to me, this dorsal shutdown response was also clear in her relationship with food. Preparing meals felt like an insurmountable task, and eating was reduced to a passive, discon-nected act—grabbing an extra chicken nugget from her kid's fast-food lunch, eating sporadically, or just grabbing an extra coffee and a chocolate bar, even when she knew it would make her feel worse. "I know I should care," she admitted, "but most days, I just don't." Her experience is a reminder that when the nervous system is stuck in survival mode, self-care can feel impossible—not because you don't want to feel better but because your body is conserving energy in the only way it knows how. Unfortunately, this survival mechanism also kept Dani from meeting her body's basic needs.

In addition to the dissociation and numbness that often accom-pany a dorsal shutdown response, I've seen a variety of ways my cli-ents experience this state while trying to improve their health. Do any of these feel familiar to you?

Difficulty Tending to Medical Needs

- Struggling to get started or follow through with health changes because it feels overwhelming
- Avoiding or postponing medical appointments, lab tests, or follow-ups
- Ignoring symptoms until they become severe
- Feeling too tired to engage with movement or daily activities
- Tuning out and dissociating from body signals such as hunger, thirst, or fatigue

Struggling with Adequate Nutrition

- Feeling like it doesn't matter what you eat—so why try?
- Ignoring hunger and fullness cues, sometimes not eating all day
- Frequent bingeing to numb out

- Eating the same foods on repeat (e.g., granola bars, toast, or frozen meals) to minimize decision fatigue
- Feeling disconnected from food choices—eating without really tasting or enjoying food

Disconnected from the Body's Needs

- Struggling to find motivation for any form of exercise—even light movement
- Feeling like even thinking about working out is exhausting
- Feeling like rest is the only thing you have the energy for, even when movement could help
- Feeling shame or guilt for not engaging in healthy behaviors, leading to more avoidance
- Thinking, "I know what to do; I just can't make myself do it"
- Believing that you'll never feel better, so what's the point in trying?

I've found that people in dorsal shutdown often *disconnect rather than take action*. However, a dorsal-driven approach to health isn't about willpower or laziness; it's about a nervous system that's overwhelmed and shutting down to conserve energy.

Diet culture also leads many into dorsal shutdown mode, especially in the face of overwhelming, contradictory nutrition advice. The Internet is saturated with conflicting opinions: Carbs are bad. No, carbs are essential. Eat six small meals a day. No, practice intermittent fasting. Dairy is inflammatory. No, dairy is a superfood. The sheer volume of competing voices, each claiming to be the definitive answer, can create decision fatigue, paralysis, and avoidance.

This is how dorsal shutdown hijacks your plate.

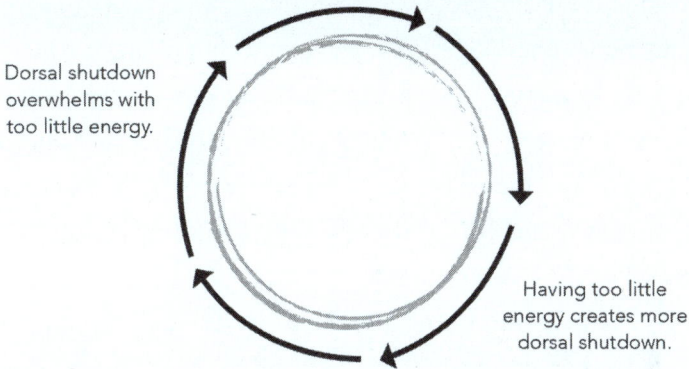

Dorsal shutdown overwhelms with too little energy.

Having too little energy creates more dorsal shutdown.

When your nervous system gets overwhelmed, it can shut down completely—making nourishment feel out of reach.

When people are bombarded with messages that make eating feel like a high-stakes test they are destined to fail, their nervous system may shift into a dorsal shutdown state—the body's way of conserving energy when stress becomes too much. This can show up as giving up on trying to eat "healthy" altogether, feeling numb or detached from food choices, skipping meals unintentionally, or relying on ultra-convenient, low-effort foods because the idea of planning, prepping, or making "the right" choice feels impossible.

Instead of fostering confidence in making nourishing decisions, diet culture erodes trust in your ability to eat intuitively, leaving many people disconnected from their needs, exhausted by the pressure, and unable to engage with food in a way that feels sustainable or supportive.

Do you resonate more with Jan's response to stress or Dani's? Maybe you experience some of each. Remember, while most of us do have a "home away from home"—a nervous system state we default to in times of stress—we are not locked into just one response. Instead, we can shift between states of ventral regulation, sympathetic activation, and dorsal shutdown many times a day.

This is why you might wake up hypermotivated, frantically researching new health protocols, reorganizing your pantry, or planning a strict wellness regimen—only to find, hours later, that you're completely exhausted, disengaged, and unable to do anything beyond sitting on the couch, scrolling on your phone, or numbing out with food or TV. These fluctuations aren't a sign of failure or inconsistency; they're simply your nervous system adapting in real time to perceived levels of stress and safety.

In my view, healthy eating is a verb, defined as meeting your body where it is—not where you think it should be. Just as I don't expect you to spend your entire life walking around in a regulated and connected state 100 percent of the time, I also don't expect that you are going to eat "healthy" 100 percent of the time. One day, you'll have the capacity to cook something healthy and nourishing for your body, and the next day you may be so anxious and overwhelmed that you order pizza. Sometimes, you'll look up recipes and execute them perfectly, and other days, you'll buy produce with good intentions but find it weeks later in the vegetable "hospice drawer" of your fridge (where your forgotten vegetables go to die).

If eating well were just about knowing what to do, everyone would be doing it. But food choices aren't made in a vacuum; they're deeply tied to energy, capacity, and safety. When the nervous system is dysregulated, even the most well-intentioned plans for "healthy eating" can feel impossible to execute. Many people assume they lack willpower or discipline when in reality, their nervous system is prioritizing survival over meal planning and food prep. I often hear people say, "I just can't make myself eat healthy," but what they're really expressing is "I haven't felt safe enough to have the energy to eat in the way I want to." And when safety is compromised—whether from stress, trauma, or depletion—the nervous system seeks relief in whatever way it can, often through behaviors that society labels as "good" or "bad" coping strategies.

Some responses, such as taking a walk, deep breathing, or meditating, are often praised as "good" or "healthy" self-care. Others, such as drinking alcohol, emotional eating, eating far past fullness, or zoning out in front of the TV for hours, tend to be judged as "bad" or "unhealthy." The image below illustrates this divide, showing culturally approved ways of coping, such as exercise, meditation, and therapy, alongside culturally stigmatized ways, such as emotional eating or zoning out.

Coping behaviors are adaptive.

Culturally Approved Ways to Get Out of a Survival State

(Often seen as universally "healthy," "productive," "self-care")

- Exercise (going for a run, yoga, lifting weights)
- Meditation and mindfulness practices
- Deep breathing techniques
- Cleaning and organizing
- Therapy or talking it out with a friend
- Journaling or creative expression
- Eating "clean" or following a specific diet
- Spending time in nature
- Cold plunges, sauna use, biohacking techniques
- Volunteering or acts of service
- Drinking herbal tea or using essential oils

Culturally Stigmatized Ways of Coping with a Survival State

(Often labeled as universally "bad," "unhealthy," "self-sabotaging")

- Drinking alcohol or using recreational substances
- Emotional eating, or eating far past fullness
- Scrolling social media or binge-watching TV
- Seeking comfort from past relationships
- Sleeping excessively or avoiding responsibilities
- Zoning out, dissociating, or numbing feelings

Whether celebrated or stigmatized, all of these behaviors are attempts to exit a survival state and regulate the nervous system.

In reality, *both* sets of behaviors emerge from the same adaptive need—to shift the nervous system out of a survival state and back toward ventral regulation. And *both* sets of behaviors have the possibility of being supportive in the moment but maladaptive in excess or over time. Don't believe me? Think about people who turn to exercise as their primary coping tool but push their bodies to the point of injury, or those who use strict dietary control to manage stress, only to develop an unhealthy relationship with food. In contrast, someone who occasionally decompresses with a glass of wine, intentionally seeks out comfort foods after a hard week, or has a night of binge-watching reality TV to help deal with a breakup may find that these strategies help them reset without negative consequences. The key difference isn't whether a behavior is labeled as "good" or "bad" by society; it's whether it truly supports ventral regulation and well-being over time.

When we begin to examine our behaviors with food through the lens of nervous system regulation rather than morality, it shifts the conversation from judgment to understanding. Instead of asking, "Is this food good or bad?" or "Am I a good or bad person for eating this?" we can start asking, "What is this food doing for me?" This perspective allows us to move beyond shame and toward curiosity—recognizing that all coping strategies, whether they are eating too much, too little, or (gasp!) fast food are adaptive responses to the situation.

So how do we start moving toward healthy eating?

In trauma work, somatic therapist Peter Levine describes a concept called **pendulation**. Pendulation describes the nervous system's ability to move between states of sympathetic activation and dorsal shutdown as it attempts to self-regulate. Said again for the people at the back, what you've interpreted as inconsistency and lack of will-power is your body pendulating back and forth between nervous system states. Rather than seeing these shifts as a sign that something is wrong, we can recognize them as the body's way of trying to restore balance.

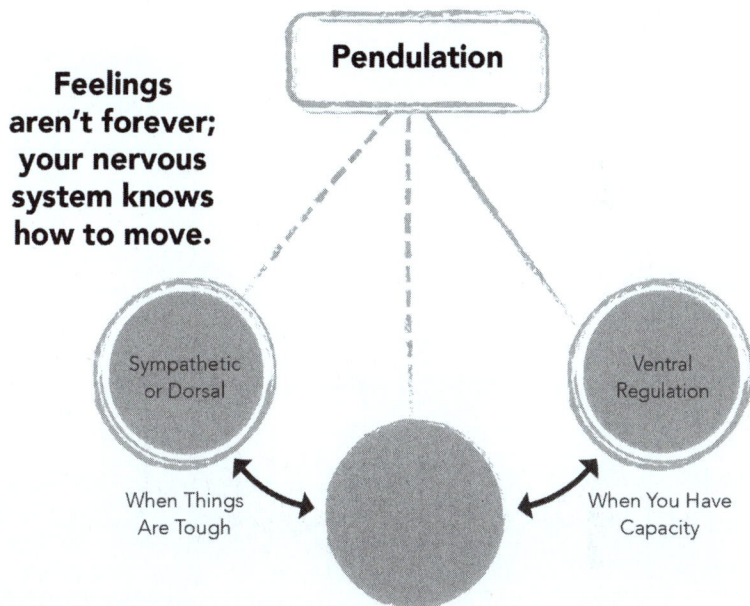

Feelings aren't forever; your nervous system knows how to move.

Pendulation

Sympathetic or Dorsal

Ventral Regulation

When Things Are Tough

When You Have Capacity

Pendulation is a sign your nervous system is working. This back-and-forth movement between regulation and survival states supports long-term healing.

When I'm with a client in session who is experiencing a survival state (which happens all the time), I might use pendulation to help their nervous systems find regulation. Sometimes, this looks like a client breaking down in tears, overwhelmed by emotions they didn't expect to surface. Other times, they shut down completely, going quiet, staring off into space, or struggling to find words. In those moments, I allow them to feel whatever they are feeling. And then, when they are ready, I'll ask them to focus on a sensation that feels safe, such as the feeling of their feet on the floor or the chair supporting them. We may shift back and forth a couple of times between the distressing and neutral sensations, allowing their nervous system to experience movement (pendulation) rather than staying stuck. Over time, practicing moving in and out of survival states can help remind our nervous systems and brains that feelings aren't forever and that what we're experiencing in this moment isn't permanent.

Pendulation can also happen when you're trying to change your food habits. When you're well-regulated and grounded, you might delight in making meals from scratch or enjoying long, lazy meals at your local Italian restaurant, or you may go get ice cream with the kids and enjoy every single bite. In a survival state, you might not eat at all, eat in the car, put in an emergency takeout order, largely exist on protein bars, or eat in a way that doesn't match your health goals.

When you're able to recognize that your food choices are adaptive acts of self-care rather than "bad habits," it shifts the narrative from shame (a survival state in and of itself) to empowerment.

In my head, I can hear some of you saying that your approach to food during hard times is all fast food and processed junk and that under no circumstances should you "allow yourself" to go back there. I'd follow up with a couple questions. First, is it always possible for you to eat in a way you believe is healthy during a survival state? Second, if you *do* manage to eat in that way, is it creating more wear and tear on your nervous system due to the rigidity of the demands? Put another way, is forcing yourself to "eat healthy" causing you even more stress during an already stressed time?

If so, is that really your best bet? What if, instead of feeling like we have to keep up our own standards when we're underwater, we just give permission to feed ourselves in whatever ways feel possible while emphasizing ways that get us back into ventral regulation? Might the care you've just given to your nervous system by responding to its needs by not overly stressing yourself get you back to feeling centered faster? As the saying often used for babies reminds us, "Fed is best."

Healthy Eating Is Adaptive Eating

Traditional Western models of healthy eating often revolve around rigid rules, external guidelines, and moralized food choices, reinforcing the idea that eating healthy means following a set plan perfectly. But for people who have experienced trauma, or who struggle with nervous system dysregulation, these strict approaches often backfire—either triggering sympathetic activation and over-control (hyperfixation on "perfect" eating) or dorsal shutdown (avoidance, paralysis, or giving up).

A trauma-informed approach to eating looks different. Instead of forcing yourself to follow rigid food rules no matter how you feel, ask, "Where is my nervous system right now? What kind of support do I need?"

When you're in a ventral state—feeling regulated, safe, and connected—it's much easier to make intentional, nutritious food choices. You might enjoy meal planning, trying new foods, or tuning into hunger and fullness cues naturally.

But when you're stuck in a survival state—sympathetic activation or dorsal shutdown—your nervous system is busy trying to protect you. Long-term goals, mindful eating, and flexible food choices aren't easily available.

		What is possible in a survival state	What is possible in regulation
Ventral regulation allows choice.	**Responding well to hunger and fullness cues**	No	Yes
	Prioritizing long-term needs and goals	No	Yes
	Choosing foods that balance nutrition and enjoyment	No	Yes

When regulation is present, your full range of food choices opens up. When you're in survival, the goal shifts to getting through this moment.

At this point, it should be clear: Eating well isn't just about knowing what to do—it's about whether your nervous system feels safe enough to do it.

If you've ever struggled to stick to a nutrition plan, felt ashamed for grabbing fast food after a hard day, or blamed yourself for not cooking the beautiful meals you planned, I hope you can see it's not a failure. Learning to feed yourself in a way that matches your current capacity is one of the most radical, trauma-informed acts of self-care there is.

When we honor where our nervous system is—whether we're activated, shut down, or regulated—we can begin to make food choices that actually support healing rather than add more stress. Adaptive eating isn't rigid. It's flexible, compassionate, and grounded in meeting your body where it is today.

But food choices don't exist in a vacuum; they are deeply shaped by the people around us. In the next chapter, we'll explore how family, friends, and culture shape our relationship with food—often in ways we don't even realize—and how understanding those influences can free us to build a more peaceful, supportive relationship with healthy eating.

CHAPTER 3

Where Did My Relationship with Food Go Wrong?

We don't learn to hate our bodies or moralize our food choices in a vacuum. We're taught.

—Christy Harrison, MPH, RD, *Anti-Diet*

For many of us, food isn't just about staying fed—it's about connection. It shows up at birthdays and breakups, holidays and quiet weeknights, often bringing people together when words fall short. Whether it's cooking for someone you love or passing a dish across the table, food becomes a way to express care, build closeness, and share moments that matter.

For some, food really is a love language all its own.

One of the best examples of this was how my cousin Abbey and her family navigated nutrition during the cancer recurrence of her eleven-year-old son, Sam. In a Facebook post updating friends and family, my cousin mentioned a planned trip to Five Guys, one of Sam's favorite restaurants. Someone made an unfortunate comment referencing how they really shouldn't eat fast food if they wanted Sam to recover.

Abbey doesn't remember this comment specifically, but she shared that many people provided so much unsolicited nutrition advice that it all blended together. I'm going to give you her words here because I think they do a better job than I ever could talking about how food can strengthen relationships and bring healing:

> Cancer took away so much of Sam's autonomy and the pleasant things he usually enjoyed. Food became that one bright spot of something he could look forward to and the one thing that could be entirely of his choosing.
>
> Sam's cancer treatment was a ninety-minute drive each way, and time at the clinic itself could stretch into an all-day affair. Occasionally, he had to fast starting the night before, and sometimes an outpatient clinic day would end with an unexpected inpatient admission. It could be quite grueling, so Sam being able to eat out at the end of the day felt like a victory celebration.
>
> Mike [Sam's dad] was often the one who took him to the clinic, and he would have Sam pick a place to go out to eat before they headed home. Sam usually opted for one of two places: Five Guys

(because he loved cheeseburgers) or a local mom-and-pop called Oriental Cafe. The staff at Oriental Cafe grew to know Sam, and he felt welcome there. Our family rarely ate out, so this was definitely a mood lifter for him.

Allowing Sam to choose what he wanted to eat was also one of the ways we could express our love and empathy as his parents. No request was too extreme, so though the clinic staff would tell us it was difficult to find restaurants that would deliver to the hospital, we'd still manage to find a place open at 10 PM that would deliver the Chinese food Sam had requested. He asked very little of us, so we jumped at any opportunity to serve him.

It was also a way for Joe and Claire [Sam's siblings] to express their love for him. We used to stop in at Trader Joe's and they'd help me pick out treats they thought or knew he liked.

I have long valued a nutritious diet, and I wanted Sam to eat the most nourishing food possible. Until he was admitted to the hospital full time after his cancer relapsed, most of what he ate was what I cooked at home. But I thought that his morale was equally important to his nutrition in fighting cancer, so I made space for him also to eat what he wanted.

Sam passed away a few years before I shifted careers to become a nutrition provider, but I never forgot the feeling of reading Abbey's powerful words, and I have always tried to acknowledge the many roles food plays in healing.

Unfortunately, while food can be a source of comfort, connection, and even healing, it can also cause harm. Sometimes, that harm is unintentional—well-meaning advice that instills fear rather than support, rigid food rules that disconnect us from our own needs, or cultural messages that reduce food to a moral choice of "good" or "bad." And sometimes, our drive to stay connected to others—especially early caregivers or important relationships—shapes our food patterns in ways we don't even realize.

When We Choose Attachment over Authenticity

Jamie was ten the first time she started hiding snacks. Her mom was chronically on a diet and often made critical comments about other people's food choices. "Your grandmother certainly didn't need that piece of cake after dinner," she'd say with a tight smile. But it wasn't until Jamie reached the early stages of puberty that her mom's food judgment started to turn toward her. Suddenly, whenever Jamie asked for seconds, her mom would pause and say, "Oh, honey . . . are you really still hungry?"

From then on, Jamie learned to read her mom's body language before reaching for a second helping or even a snack. She began to measure her bites at dinner. She praised her mom's dieting efforts, even mimicking them. Every time she'd feel hungry, she would push down that feeling with the knowledge that her mom wouldn't think it was "right." Eventually, Jamie's body became something to manage and her hunger something to doubt. The discomfort of her hunger paled in comparison to the discomfort of disappointing her mom.

Unfortunately, Jamie's experience is not unique. Many children learn to prioritize staying connected to their caregivers over listening to their own bodies. When faced with a choice between honoring internal cues—such as hunger, fullness, or emotional needs—and preserving a sense of closeness or approval from a parent, children will almost always choose connection. It's not a conscious decision but a survival response.

As Gabor Maté describes it, this is the dynamic of "attachment over authenticity"—the idea that to maintain attachment, a child may silence or override their own inner experience. Over time, this trade-off can disconnect a person from their body's signals, laying the groundwork for disordered eating patterns that begin in childhood.

Why We Choose Attachment over Authenticity (Especially with Food)

From an early age, our deepest instinct isn't to be fully ourselves; it's to stay connected. That means we often learn to hide or shut down parts of who we are to keep relationships intact. This instinct doesn't just shape how we act—it also shapes how we eat.

Here's what the research shows:

- Connection comes first. When we don't feel safe to be ourselves, authenticity takes a backseat. That includes food. You may override your hunger, avoid asking for what you want, or try to eat "perfectly" to gain approval.[1]

- Your nervous system remembers. When attachment is shaky, your body may default into survival mode—sympathetic activation or dorsal shutdown. This affects how you experience hunger, fullness, and safety around food.[2]

- Parts of you go into hiding. According to Internal Family Systems (IFS), we often tuck away the parts of us that feel shame, or that were rejected—such as the part that wanted to enjoy food or speak up about what it needed. Healing involves inviting those parts back into connection.[3]

- How you bond matters. Attachment styles—formed in childhood but active in adulthood—have a big impact on mental health, including how we manage stress, emotions, and self-care.[4]
- Attachment trauma runs deep. When the person we're supposed to turn to for comfort is also the source of distress, it leaves a lasting imprint on the nervous system and body. This kind of trauma affects everything: how we eat, how we relate, and how we self-regulate.[4]

As psychotherapist Jon Allen writes, "Attachment trauma is the overwhelming experience of feeling alone in the midst of an unbearable emotional state or realizing that the attachment person itself is the cause of overwhelming distress."[4]

Even in homes without obvious "big T" food trauma, a caregiver's complicated relationship with food can ripple down through small, everyday moments: a mother casually labeling foods as "good" or "bad," a father joking that you have to "earn" dessert, a grandparent looking uncomfortable if you didn't clean your plate. These moments might seem minor or forgettable on the surface, but to a child, they send powerful messages about what's acceptable, lovable, or safe. And those messages don't just land in your mind. They land in your body. Over time, your nervous system stores them as part of its internal map, linking food not just to nourishment but to approval, shame, and belonging.

When authenticity—honoring what you needed—put your attachment at risk, you adapted. You stayed quiet. You made your needs smaller. You said, "I'm fine," when you weren't. Over time, that survival strategy can harden into patterns such as chronic dieting, binge-restrict cycles, emotional eating, or simply feeling disconnected from your body's cues.

This isn't a character flaw. It's an adaptation your nervous system made to protect you.

And unless we actively work to change it, that adaptation follows us into adulthood.

Food-related attachment challenges don't end when we grow up. They show up later too: A partner who eats "clean" and makes you feel guilty for your choices. A friend who jokes about "sugar addiction" just as you unwrap a candy bar. A doctor who hands you a restrictive diet plan that feels unsafe, but you feel too intimidated to question it. So you stay quiet. You push down the voice inside that says, "This doesn't feel right," because approval still feels like safety.

After escaping an emotionally abusive relationship, Sofia found herself unable to eat without immense anxiety. Her ex had criticized her weight, controlled what she ate, and shamed her for indulging in anything "unhealthy." Even after their breakup, the echoes of his voice lingered in her mind. She tried to avoid eating in front of others and became fixated on "clean" eating, her nervous system still bracing for judgment. Though she knew logically that food wasn't dangerous, her reactions told a different story.

This scenario—where a partner dictates or judges your food choices—is so common in my group nutrition practice that, behind the scenes, my team has a running joke: "Dump him and eat a snack." We'd never say it to a client, of course—but we wish we could.

When food has been tied to punishment, reward, or moral judgment, the simple act of eating can become loaded with shame, guilt, or anxiety. But food is not something we have to earn.

Trauma disrupts attachment at the roots. Whether through neglect, abuse, emotional inconsistency, or emotional unavailability, trauma teaches the body that safety is conditional, that love must be earned, that needs should be hidden, delayed, or denied.

These early wounds don't just shape how we relate to caregivers. They shape how we relate to ourselves—and to food:

- **Anxious Attachment.** When your early needs were met inconsistently—sometimes cared for, sometimes ignored— you learned to stay hyperattuned to others' reactions. You may use food to self-soothe, manage anxiety, or seek approval through appearance and body size. Eating can become a way to regulate relationships: "If I look a certain way, maybe I'll be loved." The focus often stays outward—on pleasing others— rather than inward, on what your body actually needs.

- **Avoidant Attachment.** When your needs were regularly unmet or dismissed, you learned that vulnerability wasn't safe. You may suppress hunger cues, downplay the importance of food, or avoid eating in front of others as a way to stay in control. Nourishment—both emotional and physical—can feel threatening, so you might push it away, convincing yourself you don't really need it. Independence becomes a shield, even when your body is asking for care.

- **Disorganized Attachment.** If your caregivers were both a source of safety and fear—loving one moment and frightening the next—your nervous system may struggle to create a coherent pattern around eating. Food behaviors might swing dramatically: restricting, bingeing, avoiding food, or obsessing over it without clear reason. Eating can feel confusing and chaotic, as if your body's hunger and fullness signals are unpredictable or untrustworthy. Safety feels elusive, and food becomes another place where you brace for the unexpected.

In each case, the food behavior makes perfect sense when viewed through the lens of attachment: it's not a failure—it's a survival strategy, carried forward into adult life. Healing isn't about forcing yourself to eat perfectly or rejecting your past. It starts by noticing, paying attention to the ways your body and nervous system respond in different situations. When you feel that pull to abandon your own needs—whether it's eating a food that doesn't feel good to your body just to avoid conflict, or skipping meals to stay invisible—pause and get curious. What state is your nervous system in? Are you reaching for attachment at the cost of your authenticity? Naming these moments is powerful. It gives you the first glimpse of choice: the chance to stay connected to yourself even when old patterns suggest otherwise.

When Restriction Brings Control

For Bea, a college junior diagnosed with IBS-D, food quickly shifted from nourishment to obsession. What started as a well-meaning recommendation from her nurse practitioner to follow a low-FODMAP diet soon spiraled. When her symptoms didn't improve immediately, Bea didn't blame the plan; she blamed herself. She doubled down, eliminating more and more foods, believing that if she could just find and avoid the "right" triggers, she could finally feel safe in her body again.

By the time she arrived at my office, Bea was eating fewer than ten foods. She was terrified that adding anything else back would cause unbearable symptoms. Even foods she intellectually knew were safe triggered anxiety. I still remember a session where Bea agreed to eat a grape (something she deemed "safe") but visibly panicked when I suggested trying a raisin—a food that is, after all, just a dried grape.

Her nervous system wasn't reacting to logic. It was reacting to the overwhelming survival signal that said, "New foods are dangerous."

Bea is far from alone. Many of my clients arrive believing that restriction will save them. Sometimes it starts with physical symptoms—gut issues, allergies, chronic illness—and sometimes it starts with emotional overwhelm. Either way, restriction becomes a survival strategy: a way to create certainty, control, and safety in a world or a body that feels unpredictable.

Why Restriction Feels So Powerful

Severely restricting food can initially feel calming because it reduces the number of unpredictable sensations the body has to process. But over time, it actually stresses the HPA axis (the body's stress-response system), leading to worsened digestion, increased anxiety, and even more disconnection from hunger, fullness, and body trust.

In today's culture, this pattern gets reinforced constantly. We are praised for cutting out sugar, gluten, carbs, dairy—you name it—as if "purity" is the same as health. Discipline is glorified. Flexibility is seen as weakness. And so the nervous system—already searching for a lifeline—grabs onto the only thing it feels it can control: *less.*

Less food. Less variety. Less risk.

But ironically, the longer restriction goes on, the more fragile and reactive the body becomes. Limited diets weaken the gut microbiome, decrease tolerance to new foods, and increase both physical and emotional sensitivity to change. The very strategy meant to create safety ends up deepening fear.

When a client is stuck in this survival loop of restriction, my job isn't to tear down the walls overnight. It's to help them recognize that *this restriction isn't who they are. It's what their nervous system has been doing to try to protect them.*

Rather than pushing them to immediately reintroduce dozens of new foods, I start somewhere much more important: the nervous system's story about safety.

We ask:

- What sensations come up when you even think about eating something new?
- Where does that fear live in your body?
- Can you notice the difference between true physical danger and the nervous system's protective alarm?

Sometimes the work looks like adding one new food every few weeks. Sometimes it's simply sitting with the *idea* of a new food without acting on it, letting the nervous system process the possibility without pressure.

If you're noticing this pattern within yourself—feeling stuck in restriction but wanting more freedom—you don't have to change everything overnight. In fact, you shouldn't. Healing happens little by little, through movements your nervous system can actually tolerate.

Sometimes, that movement looks like eating just two more grapes than you normally would. Sometimes it's adding a tiny sprinkle of a new herb or spice to a dish you already feel safe eating. I've even had a client start by changing the brand of her usual pineapple juice—that was the maximum change her nervous system could handle without slipping into survival mode.

This is the true goal of healing from restriction: finding a way to expand your diet that feels possible within ventral regulation—not so overwhelming that it sends you into sympathetic activation or dorsal shutdown. Every small step you take toward variety, flexibility, and trust matters. And every step counts.

For Bea, healing didn't come from another rigid list of "safe" versus "unsafe" foods. It came from gently expanding her diet at a pace that honored her nervous system's capacity. It came from learning to name when survival energy was driving her choices. And most importantly, it came from understanding that true healing doesn't happen through perfection; it happens through flexibility, curiosity, and trust.

When Food Becomes Too Painful

Trauma doesn't have to be directly related to food or body image to profoundly impact your relationship with food.

For Lydia, fifty-four, food had once been a source of joy—weekend pancakes with her daughter, baking cookies for the holidays, and sharing meals together after a long day. But after her nineteen-year-old daughter was murdered by her boyfriend—now serving a life sentence—food became unbearable.

In the early weeks after the funeral, Lydia barely ate. Friends and family dropped off casseroles, but she let them pile up in the fridge, uneaten. Hunger came in waves, but she ignored it, unable to summon the energy to eat. When she did eat, it was mechanical—grabbing a protein bar or crackers, just enough to keep going. Within three months, she had lost fifteen pounds.

What shocked her most wasn't the weight loss itself; it was how many people *congratulated* her on it. In passing, a coworker from a different branch of her company told her she looked great. A neighbor who lived down the block, oblivious to her pain, asked what she was doing differently. Each comment felt like a slap, and she wondered how the world continued as if nothing had happened.

As the months wore on, her eating stayed all over the place. Some days, nothing sounded good, and she skipped meals without meaning to. Other days, she reached for takeout and snacks just to fill the silence, barely noticing the taste. Even the meals that once brought her joy—her daughter's favorite spaghetti, the birthday cake they used to bake together—now felt like too much to face.

Lydia's experience is a stark reminder that food is never just about calories or nutrients. It carries meaning, memory, and emotion. Grief can make eating feel impossible, or it can push us toward comfort foods in search of solace. Neither response is wrong—both are simply the body's way of coping with the unbearable.

When clients like Lydia struggle to eat after loss, I don't start with meal plans or nutrition goals. Instead, I ask, "What feels safe? What foods, if any, still hold neutral or positive associations?" Healing isn't about forcing normalcy; it's about gently rebuilding a connection to food that feels possible.

For Lydia, the first step wasn't sitting down at the table to eat a full meal, something she and her daughter used to do regularly. That felt unbearable, too closely tied to memories of their shared dinners. Instead, she found ways to eat that didn't require sitting with her grief.

I encouraged her to start by eating while driving on her way to and from work, letting the distraction of the road make food feel less overwhelming. Then, she began ordering takeout—foods she wouldn't have cooked at home, meals that didn't remind her of what she had lost. Eventually, she gave up on the thought of cooking altogether. The act of preparing meals had once been a way to care for her daughter, and without that purpose, it felt empty. Instead, she stocked her fridge with premade meals from the grocery store, things she could grab without thinking too much.

Some days, she only ate standing at the kitchen counter. Other days, she grazed on snacks rather than eat a full meal. By traditional standards, these habits might seem disorganized or even disordered, but in reality, they were a survival strategy. Eating in any way that felt possible became a bridge between total disconnection and the slow return to nourishment. Healing wasn't about forcing herself back into old routines; it was about honoring what felt doable in the moment.

How Trauma Impacts Eating

Trauma changes everything—including the way we eat.

Trauma is a major risk factor for developing eating disorders, which are serious mental illnesses that can deeply impair daily life. Research suggests that anywhere from 54 percent to 100 percent of women with eating disorders have a history of trauma.[5] But it's not just about diagnosable eating disorders. Trauma can also shape a whole spectrum of disordered eating behaviors—patterns that may not meet clinical criteria but still disrupt someone's relationship with food, body, and self.

All Eating Disorders Involve Disordered Eating, but Not All Disordered Eating Is an Eating Disorder

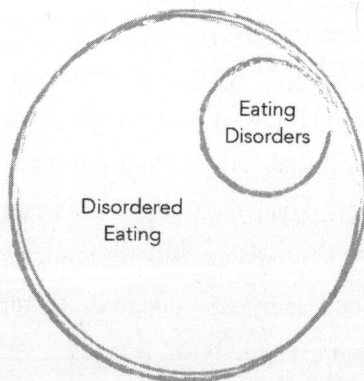

Eating Disorders

Disordered Eating

Disordered Eating: A broad term used to describe irregular eating behaviors that may not meet the diagnostic criteria for an eating disorder but still negatively affect a person's physical or emotional well-being.

Eating Disorders: A diagnosable mental health condition characterized by severe disturbances in eating behaviors and related thoughts and emotions. Eating disorders are recognized in the DSM-5 and typically require professional treatment.

Recognizing disordered eating, even if it's not a full-blown eating disorder, is the first step toward healing your relationship with food.

If you've ever struggled with an eating disorder, working with a therapist and a nutrition provider who specializes in eating disorder care is essential.

If cost is a barrier, *Project Heal* is a national nonprofit that can help. They offer free daily online meal support groups available to everyone, regardless of income, and one-on-one therapy and nutrition counseling at no cost for individuals who qualify based on financial need.

Find Project Heal online at https://www.theprojectheal.org/.

One study of young adults in the United States found that those who had experienced multiple forms of childhood or complex trauma were nearly twice as likely to report disordered eating behavior compared to those without a history of trauma.[6] When the nervous system is stuck in survival mode—whether due to childhood adversity, a single traumatic event, complex trauma, or prolonged and chronic stress—it searches for ways to regulate. For many, food becomes an accessible tool for coping. Some people develop rigid food rules, obsessing about eating "clean" as a way to create a sense of control. Others may swing between bingeing, emotional eating, and chronic dieting, their bodies desperately trying to find a sense of safety.

Regardless of where someone falls on the spectrum of disordered eating to eating disorder, trauma-informed care is essential in addressing the underlying dysregulation rather than simply focusing on the food behaviors themselves. Food is never just about food; it's often a reflection of a deeper need for safety, stability, and ventral regulation.

One way trauma contributes to disordered eating is through neuroceptive mismatches, when the nervous system misinterprets signals about the safety or danger of food. This can happen in two ways:

- **False safety.** The nervous system feels safe with food behaviors that are actually harmful. For example, Olivia, an eight-year-old with ADHD, grew up in a household where processed foods were completely banned. Her father, newly trained as a health coach, enforced a strict, restrictive diet, believing it would help her focus. In reality, it was his nervous system that felt falsely safe in control and restriction—missing the fact that these rigid rules were harming Olivia. At a friend's birthday party, she was found hiding in a closet, secretly eating cupcakes. Instead of recognizing the danger of deprivation, her father doubled down on restriction, unknowingly reinforcing disordered eating patterns such as secrecy and bingeing.

- **False danger.** The nervous system feels threatened by foods that are actually safe. This was Bea's experience. After struggling with IBS-D, Bea restricted her diet so severely that she ended up eating fewer than ten foods. Her body could have tolerated more variety, but her nervous system stayed stuck in fear, treating new foods as a threat—even when they posed no real risk.

Mismatched Neuroception

False Safety

- ⌇ Extreme restriction feels calming and "safe," even as it causes malnutrition or worsens symptoms.

- ⌇ Skipping meals feels like an achievement rather than a risk to energy and metabolism.

- ⌇ Overexercising without eating enough feels virtuous rather than depleting.

- ⌇ Following rigid, extreme diets (e.g., juice cleanses, fasts) feels like control rather than dysregulation.

- ⌇ Ignoring hunger cues feels strong or disciplined, even when it increases bingeing later.

- ⌇ Valuing external praise for weight loss or "willpower" even when it comes at the cost of health and well-being.

False Danger

- ⌇ Fear of whole food groups (such as carbs, fats, or dairy) even when there is no medical reason.

- ⌇ Anxiety about eating previously tolerated foods after receiving diet advice.

- ⌇ Panicking over small dietary changes (e.g., switching brands, trying a new spice) even when they're unlikely to cause harm.

- ⌇ Avoiding social eating situations because of fear that "unsafe" foods will be present.

- ⌇ Believing any deviation from a "perfect" diet will cause immediate health collapse.

- ⌇ Avoiding nourishing foods (such as fruits, vegetables, or grains) due to rigid food fear learned from past diet culture or health scares.

This chart shows how trauma can distort our sense of safety around food, making harmful behaviors feel "safe" and nourishing foods feel threatening.

Neuroceptive mismatches like these are at the root of many struggles with food. And this is why advice like "just eat normally" or "stop restricting" often falls flat. When someone's nervous system is responding to past survival needs—not present reality—logic alone isn't enough to create change.

For Olivia, eating forbidden foods in secret became a way to protect herself. For Bea, restriction felt like survival, even as it left her more vulnerable. Their behaviors weren't failures of willpower; they were adaptations their bodies made to survive overwhelming experiences. And healing them takes time, patience, and nervous system regulation—not just nutrition education.

The heart of trauma-informed care is recognizing that food behaviors are often survival strategies, not choices.

Healing your relationship with food isn't about forcing yourself to "do better" overnight. It's about building safety—both in the foods you eat and in how your body perceives those foods. It means moving slowly, respecting your nervous system's signals, and allowing small, manageable shifts that rebuild trust, one step at a time.

Create Gentle Movement

One of the first steps toward healing isn't forcing major food changes; it's creating gentle movement. And when I say movement, I don't mean exercise. I mean softening the rigid patterns that trauma often wraps around food.

Gentle movement helps tell your nervous system that it's safe to explore, that it's safe to stretch a little, without demanding perfection or inviting overwhelm.

You don't have to change everything all at once. In fact, trying to force big shifts when your nervous system is stuck in survival mode can backfire, making things feel even harder. Instead, start with what already feels doable, even just a little bit safe, and build from there. Pick one small food shift that feels okay, and try it from a place of ventral regulation, not pressure. Then, when you're ready, you can add something new—only if it feels like a gentle stretch, not a stress. Anchor your experiment in ventral regulation, then add a twist of something new.

Some examples of gentle movement might be the following:

- **Change a portion size slightly.** Move from one quarter cup to one third cup of a food you already tolerate, allowing yourself to honor hunger rather than sticking to an old "ideal portion" learned from a parent or diet culture.

- **Allow yourself to eat a little earlier or later than your usual schedule.** If you have rigid rules around when you eat, moving your normal eating time by just two to three minutes might give your nervous system a possible stretch that isn't an overt stress.
- **Try a small variation of a familiar food.** Try switching from plain white rice to lightly seasoned rice, brown rice, or even just a different brand, giving yourself permission to explore preference rather than sticking to only "approved" foods.
- **Eat in a different setting.** Try sitting at the table instead of standing at the counter, or eat with a trusted friend instead of eating alone if old patterns made food a private, secretive act.
- **Choose a food you enjoy even if it wasn't valued or allowed growing up.** Have a dessert you actually love instead of forcing yourself to eat only "healthy treats" to meet someone else's standards.

Each small shift signals to your nervous system that change can happen safely. And even tiny shifts matter—because every time you try something new without overwhelming your system, you're reinforcing neuroplasticity.

Neuroplasticity is the brain's ability to change and create new pathways based on experience. When you practice small, safe changes, you are literally helping your brain and body learn that food and flexibility are not threats. Over time, these tiny experiences create bigger and bigger changes in how you feel about eating.

Yes, at times this process may feel slow. You might wish you could "fix" things faster. That's normal too. But lasting healing doesn't happen through pressure or force—it's built through repetition, safety, and trust, one small, regulated step at a time.

Use External and Internal Cues to Help Regulate Eating

When we're experiencing neuroceptive mismatches, it can be difficult to feel regulated around food. If hunger signals aren't coming through clearly, or if they feel dysregulated, using external and internal strategies can help bridge the gap, giving your nervous system the structure it needs while still allowing for flexibility.

Below are some ways to support your body in finding a rhythm with food that feels both intentional and compassionate.

- **Set alarms on your phone.** A strong survival response can cause you to lose track of time, so setting alarms on your phone can help remind you of meal and snack times. If you're getting regular cues to eat, alarms on your phone can give you an intentional cue to tune in and see if you are actually hungry. Pro tip: Choose an alarm sound that isn't super jarring to your system.

- **Pre-portion snacks.** When you have a little more capacity, set up easy-to-reach snacks in small containers or bags on the counter or in the door of the refrigerator, creating a visual cue that encourages you to grab a bite.

- **Pair eating with an existing routine.** Pair meals or snacks with a habit you already do regularly, such as having breakfast after your morning shower, a snack before walking the dog, or dinner while you watch a favorite show. Yes, you read that right: I'm all in favor of using distraction (watching television) if it helps increase your ability to eat in the moment.

- **Identify alternative hunger cues.** One of my favorite clients used to tell me that when she was stressed, the only way she'd feel hunger is when she noticed her shoulders were lodged right at her earlobes. In less-stressed times, she experienced hunger as a grumbling in her stomach, so you can imagine that this very different hunger cue took a long time for her to figure out. Are there unusual cues that you're experiencing that can help remind you to eat?

- **Are you hangry, hanguished, or have hanxiety?** Often people feel emotions such as anger, depression, or anxiety when hungry. It's worth tuning into those moments and trying to eat a snack just to see what happens.

Explore What Food Feels Like in Ventral Regulation

Unlike the doctor who once told my client that eating a single cupcake on her birthday would ruin her chances of getting healthy, I believe something very different: Foods that are often labeled "unhealthy" can absolutely be part of a nourishing life—especially when eaten from a place of ventral regulation. It's not just about *what* you eat. It's about *how* you feel when you eat it.

When your nervous system is regulated—when you feel connected, and safe—your body is better able to digest, metabolize, and enjoy food. Eating from this place of safety and connection leads to real satisfaction, not shame or guilt.

You might also experience food in blended states:

- In a **ventral regulated/sympathetic activated blend**, food might feel playful and energizing—decorating cookies at a holiday party, sharing popcorn during a lively movie night, or laughing with friends over homemade pizza.
- In a **ventral regulated/dorsal shutdown blend**, food might feel grounding and deeply comforting—sipping tea when

you're feeling reflective, eating a warm bowl of soup on a cold day, or preparing a meal that connects you to someone you love.

That same cupcake can land completely differently depending on your state. If you're eating it on your birthday, surrounded by people you love, it might feel like joy, connection, and self-trust. Your body is more likely to digest it well and leave you feeling content. But if you eat it while stressed or checked out, your system may be in survival mode—making digestion sluggish and blood sugar harder to manage, leaving you with a side of guilt or regret instead of satisfaction.

This is why comfort foods are not inherently "bad." True nourishment isn't just about the nutrients food provides—it's about how the experience nourishes your whole being, body, mind, and spirit. A healthy relationship with food includes flexibility, joy, and trust in your body's ability to handle all kinds of nourishment.

Bringing It All Together

Whatever eating patterns you find yourself facing, it's important to remember that they often aren't about food alone. They're about what happens when your nervous system loses its sense of ventral regulation—the felt experience of safety, connection, and balance.

It might be tempting to think that everyone who's in a sympathetic activation eats too little, and everyone who's in dorsal shutdown eats too much. But real life is rarely that simple. I've worked with people who barely ate when overwhelmed and others who ate more to soothe and survive. Some disconnected from food altogether; others clung to it as the only source of comfort they could find.

There's no single "right" or "wrong" response here. There's only your nervous system doing what it learned to do to help you make it through.

The goal isn't to force yourself into better food habits by sheer willpower. It's to create more moments of ventral regulation. When your body feels safe enough to soften, your hunger and fullness cues tend to recalibrate on their own. Your relationship with food often shifts—not because you're trying harder, but because you're moving from survival into a place where real choice is possible.

This process isn't instant. It doesn't follow a neat timeline. Some days, eating may still feel hard. Some days, you may find yourself defaulting to old patterns. That's okay.

The more gently you return to ventral regulation, again and again, the more trust you build with yourself—and with food.

CHAPTER 4

How Do I Choose a Way of Eating That Actually Works?

Try the most effective, least invasive approach first.

—Alyson Roux, MS, CNS, LDN, NBC-HWC

If I could change one thing about how social media influencers talk about nutrition, it would be the one-size-fits-all mindset—the assumption that what works for them will work for everyone. Statements such as "everyone should go gluten-free," "no one should eat carbs," or "you're not healthy unless you eat nine to thirteen servings of vegetables a day" oversimplify nutrition and can be misleading and often harmful. While these approaches might support one person's health, they could negatively impact someone else's.

Nutrition requires nuance—it's personal. In this chapter, we'll explore the key factors that help me and my clients determine the right nutrition approach for their unique needs, health history, and lifestyle. Below is a list of common "healthy eating" rules you've likely heard from social media influencers or in wellness circles. Before we dive in, I want to be clear—I'm *not* saying these rules define healthy eating. In fact, what's considered "healthy" depends entirely on your nervous system, your body's needs, and your circumstances.

Instead of automatically accepting or rejecting these ideas, I want you to pause and check in with your nervous system as you read through each one. Does the idea make you feel energized, motivated, or neutral? Does it bring up stress, anxiety, resistance, or overwhelm?

Pay attention to whether your body shifts into a sympathetic activation state (feeling tense, angry, or pressured to "do it perfectly") or a dorsal shutdown state (feeling hopeless, overwhelmed, or like the effort isn't worth it). Your reaction can tell you a lot about whether a particular idea is supportive or harmful *for you*.

Here are some examples of common food "rules":

- Eat vegetables with every meal.
- Avoid sugar.
- Stick to whole foods—no processed foods.
- Drink at least eight glasses of water a day.
- No eating after 8 PM.
- Limit carbs or avoid them entirely.
- Plan and meal prep every week to avoid unhealthy choices.
- Avoid drinking calories (soda, alcohol, etc.).
- Fast for at least twelve hours overnight.

If a food rule or healthy eating idea leaves you feeling overwhelmed, pressured, ashamed, or stuck, it's not supporting your health—even if it looks "healthy" on paper.

You might be thinking, *But aren't some of these rules objectively good for me?*

Maybe, but here's the crucial piece: if your nervous system perceives a rule as a threat—because it feels rigid, overwhelming, shame based, or impossible—your system will react against it, and it will feel like a struggle, no matter how logical it sounds.

Let's break it down:

- You decide to eliminate simple carbs to help support your blood sugar. At first, you feel motivated. But soon, you realize life has gotten really tough. Grocery shopping feels like a minefield. You have no idea what to eat when friends ask you to dinner. Anxiety builds every time you even think about eating a carbohydrate. Eventually, your nervous system either spikes into sympathetic activation (urgency, frustration) or collapses into dorsal shutdown (avoidance, giving up) and you're done with this well-intentioned experiment. It's not about willpower—it's a stress response.

- You try meal prepping every Sunday. You plan, list, shop, and then . . . collapse. The ongoing burden of organizing meals, prepping, and meeting high expectations triggers a survival state. You end the weekend having prepped nothing, feeling shame instead of support.

- You try to drink eight glasses of water a day. You start strong but find water boring, tasteless, or unpalatable. Frustration builds. You set reminders. You buy a fancy water bottle. You berate yourself when you forget. Eventually, you stop trying—not from laziness but because you're exhausted by the attempt.

Each of these examples shows a fundamental mismatch: Your brain's plan didn't consider your nervous system's needs. That's a failed New Year's resolution waiting to happen.

When I work with clients to figure out what a truly healthy eating plan looks like for them, we don't start by listing off food rules. We start by asking better questions—questions that take into account your body's signals, your nervous system's reactions, and what actually feels possible and supportive for you. In the next section, I'll walk you through the questions I use to help clients uncover what "healthy" looks like for them.

How Can I Eat in a Way That Supports Health and Connection?

When considering a diet change—especially one that requires more than just adding an extra serving of vegetables—it's crucial to think about how it will affect your social life.

I'm not kidding here. Food isn't just about nourishment; it's a core part of how we connect with others.

Whether it's sharing a meal with friends, celebrating a holiday with family, or grabbing coffee with a coworker, food plays a central role in our relationships. Polyvagal theory reminds us that social connection fosters ventral regulation—the state where we feel safe, engaged, and emotionally connected. Isolation, on the other hand—whether from avoiding meals with others or feeling anxious about food choices—can shift us into a survival state, pushing us into sympathetic activation or dorsal shutdown.

If your diet makes social situations feel overwhelming, forces you to constantly monitor what you *"can't"* eat, or leaves you feeling like an outsider at the table, it may do more harm than good to your overall well-being.

Let's take the example of someone with a history of trauma who now has IBS. Together with their nutrition provider, they might consider evidence-based dietary patterns such as a low-FODMAP or Mediterranean diet to ease their gut symptoms. While these evidence-based approaches can help, they also bring real-world challenges:

- Many restaurant dishes contain high-FODMAP ingredients, making dining out stressful.
- A strict Mediterranean diet might demand significant meal prep and feel difficult to maintain in group settings.

If every meal becomes a source of tension, the nervous system may shift into a survival response. You might move into sympathetic activation, feeling anxious and preoccupied with making "perfect" choices—or into dorsal shutdown, avoiding meals with others altogether because the restrictions feel too overwhelming.

Before committing to a special diet, it's helpful to pause and ask these questions:

- Will this diet allow me to share meals with friends and family?
- Do I feel comfortable modifying meals at restaurants or bringing my own food to gatherings?
- Does this way of eating help me stay connected to others, or does it push me toward isolation?
- Can I follow this approach without feeling stressed, preoccupied, or trapped in rigid thinking?

A diet that reduces symptoms but leaves you feeling lonely, disconnected, or hyperfocused on food rules may not be truly supportive in the long term. If dietary changes are cutting you off from the relationships that bring you comfort and resilience, it's worth reassessing how to modify them in a way that supports both your body and your need for connection.

Using the example of the person with IBS, a more flexible approach could honor both health needs and the nervous system's need for safety:

- If following a low-FODMAP diet, could you focus on eliminating only the biggest triggers rather than restricting everything?
- If aiming for a Mediterranean diet, could you focus on adding nourishing foods rather than stressing over what to remove?

Ultimately, the best diet isn't just the one that reduces symptoms; it's the one that also supports your ability to live fully and stay connected.

Of course, there are times when strict dietary changes are absolutely necessary. Conditions such as severe food allergies, celiac disease, or advanced kidney disease require careful adherence to protect health. But even in these situations, maintaining social engagement matters.

Here are a few ways to protect both your health and your relationships:

- Communicate your needs in advance. Let the host know about your dietary needs ahead of time and work together on a plan.
- Offer to bring a dish. That way, you know there will be something safe for you to eat—and it allows others to share the meal with you.
- Find go-to restaurant options. A little research ahead of time makes eating out feel much less stressful.
- Reframe the focus of gatherings. Center the connection

around shared activities, not just the food—like game nights, hikes, creative projects, or book clubs.

Even when food restrictions are nonnegotiable, finding ways to stay socially engaged is just as important as maintaining dietary boundaries. When choosing or adapting a special diet, the real goal isn't just symptom relief—it's nourishing your body and protecting the connections that help you thrive.

How Do I Know If a Nutrition Trend Is Actually Backed by Science?

My team and I joke—far more often than we probably should—about how easy it would be to make up a completely random food rule, declare it the next big health trend, and watch it spread online like wildfire. We imagine coming up with something totally arbitrary, such as the "Only Eat Beige Foods Before Noon" diet or the "Cucumber-First Method," where you have to take a bite of cucumber before every meal for "optimal digestion and detoxification."

And honestly? With the right hashtags and a pretty Instagram feed, it would probably catch on.

That's the frustrating part: how quickly baseless nutrition trends can spread not because they're backed by solid evidence but because they're presented with enough confidence and charisma. Meanwhile, real evidence-based recommendations—ones that honor nuance, individual differences, and context—struggle to compete with the appeal of simple, clear-cut answers.

This is exactly why we do the work we do: to help people cut through the noise and make food choices that actually support them, not just whatever happens to be trending this week (#cucumberfirst).

When considering any diet change, the most important question isn't "Is this popular?" It's "Is this backed by evidence—and right for me, right now, with the life I'm actually living?"

Before making any sweeping changes to the way you eat, it's crucial to pause and ask whether the approach is truly grounded in research—or if it's fueled by personal anecdotes, cherry-picked data, marketing hype, or a desire to sell you something.

The truth is it's really common for us to gravitate to "the sexy stuff," and unfortunately, evidence-based nutrition is rarely flashy. It's not about extreme cleanses, rigid elimination diets, or overnight miracles. Good nutrition tends to be slow, steady, adaptable—and often a little boring compared to the viral trends promising instant transformation.

But boring is good. Boring means sustainable. Boring means it actually works.

Take Liam, a seven-year-old boy with ADHD who came to work with one of my interns after first seeing a local dietitian. Instead of starting with practical, evidence-based strategies—such as boosting protein intake; adding foods rich in antioxidants such as blueberries, grapes, and cocoa; or increasing omega-3 fats from fish, flax, and walnuts to support brain health—the dietitian immediately recommended a six-food elimination diet and an aggressive gut antimicrobial supplement protocol.

This advice wasn't based on lab results, gut symptoms, or any objective evidence. Instead, the provider made sweeping claims—without scientific support—that "everyone with ADHD has gut dysbiosis" and that "bad bacteria" needed to be "killed" to improve focus.

To be fair, research does show that gut health can influence cognitive function, and in some cases, gut imbalances may play a role in ADHD symptoms.[1] I've worked with clients where a careful, targeted gut approach—sometimes including short-term eliminations or herbal antimicrobials—made a real difference in focus, mood, and well-being.

But these interventions are never my starting point, and they should never be applied as a blanket solution, especially not for kids. They require a clear clinical reason, careful assessment, and a plan for reintroducing foods and supporting the microbiome in a sustainable way.

With Liam, the outcome was sadly predictable. His parents struggled to find enough foods he would eat on the prescribed restrictive diet. Meals became a battle, social events became stressful, and instead of improving, Liam's focus got worse.

Rather than starting with simple, evidence-based steps—such as increasing omega-3s or adding antioxidant-rich foods—his family was pulled into a stressful, unnecessary protocol that drained their energy and added disruption to daily life.

The real issue wasn't just that the intervention failed; it was that it wasted time and attention that could have gone toward strategies that actually work. Good nutrition often doesn't look flashy. It's small, steady, sustainable changes—the kind that build real health, even if they don't go viral on Instagram.

Let's take another example. Imagine you're experiencing bloating and digestive discomfort. A quick search online might lead you to a variety of conflicting advice—some people say to go gluten-free, others recommend cutting out dairy, and some influencers might tell you to eliminate lectins, nightshades, or even all grains. But what actually has scientific support?

If you work with a knowledgeable certified nutrition specialist (CNS) or registered dietitian (RD), they're not going to immediately jump straight to a specific diet. They'll ask a ton of questions first—about your medical history, current diagnoses, symptoms, lifestyle, and personal goals—and use that information, along with the latest scientific research, to guide their suggestions. They *might* suggest a low-FODMAP diet, or they *might* lean toward a Mediterranean-style plan. They might also go a completely different direction because they have realized that you're reacting to a specific food. Either way, their guidance will be tailored to *you*, not a one-size-fits-all list of food rules.

Before making a significant change to your diet, consider these key factors:

Is There High-Quality Research to Support It?

A strong nutrition recommendation is backed by well-conducted studies, not just one-off findings or personal testimonials. This is the type of evidence we find in systematic reviews, meta-analyses, or randomized controlled trials (RCTs) in peer-reviewed journals. If an approach is based only on anecdotes, personal experience, or a single small study, be skeptical.

In a world where nutrition advice spreads faster than ever, knowing how to verify claims is essential. If you hear about a diet trend, a food intervention for a specific disease, or a study someone mentioned online, take a moment to investigate before accepting it as truth.

One of the best ways to do this is by using AI to do some of the heavy lifting—while still prioritizing evidence-based sources. You can ask your favorite AI tool to search for high-quality research by requesting direct website citations from PubMed or other reputable medical databases. Be specific: Ask for RCTs, systematic reviews, or meta-analyses, which sit at the top of the evidence hierarchy and carry more scientific weight than anecdotal reports or small case studies.

Sample AI query: "Find peer-reviewed research studies from PubMed that examine the effects of plant-based diets on anxiety. Please include only meta-analyses, systematic reviews, or randomized controlled trials, and provide direct links to the studies."

Once you find a study that looks promising, copy and paste the abstract or key findings back into the AI tool and ask it to summarize the study in clear, readable language—perhaps even in bullet points. This helps you quickly grasp the main takeaways without having to decode dense scientific jargon.

To go even further, ask AI to evaluate the strength of the evidence in the study by explaining the statistics given. Was it a large, well-designed study or a small, preliminary trial? Did the results show a strong effect, or were they inconclusive? Understanding the quality of the research helps you determine whether the claim is truly backed by science—or if it's just hype.

Who Is Promoting It, and What Is Their Motive?

What is the educational background of the person pushing this approach? Are they trying to sell a product, book, or supplement line? Or perhaps they are trying to sell an idea that doesn't sit well with your nervous system. Always consider the source.

Does It Offer a One-Size-Fits-All Solution?

A red flag in any nutrition advice is the claim that "everyone should" follow a specific diet. Humans are incredibly diverse—our genetics, microbiomes, health conditions, and lifestyles all play a role in what works best for us. A good approach should be adaptable and consider individual needs.

By considering these factors, you can make more informed decisions about your nutrition, avoiding misinformation while confidently choosing food strategies that are supported by real evidence.

Does This Change Put Me at Risk for Nutrient Deficiencies or Insufficiencies?

When considering a new dietary approach, it's easy to focus on what you're removing—cutting out sugar, eliminating dairy, going keto, or swearing off gluten. But what's often overlooked is what you might be losing nutritionally in the process. Any restrictive diet, even one with a solid evidence base, has the potential to create nutritional gaps if it's not carefully planned.

The goal of any dietary shift should be to support your health, not unintentionally create new issues. If a diet improves one area—such as reducing bloating or stabilizing blood sugar—but leaves you fatigued, struggling with brain fog, or losing hair because you aren't finding enough foods to eat, it's not actually serving you.

Before committing to a major dietary change, ask yourself:

- Am I removing entire food groups? If so, am I replacing those nutrients with alternative sources?
- Does this approach provide enough calories and nutrients to sustain my daily energy needs?
- Am I at risk of key nutrient deficiencies? For example:
  - If I'm cutting out dairy, where will I get calcium and vitamin D?

- If I'm eliminating grains, am I getting enough fiber, B vitamins, and iron?
- If I'm avoiding animal products, am I ensuring adequate intake of vitamin B12, iron, and omega-3s?
- Do I feel physically well on this diet? Am I experiencing low energy, lightheadedness, poor digestion, or any other warning signs of nutritional inadequacy?

Let's take the example of eliminating gluten.

Thirty-five years ago, after my mom was first diagnosed with celiac disease (CD), she ordered a gluten-free meal on a plane. Amazingly, the airline did provide a gluten-free option—but had clearly provided little training to the flight attendants since one loudly asked, "Who ordered the glutton-free meal?" (Yes, you read that correctly.) These days, I doubt there's anyone who hasn't heard of someone going gluten-free.

There's a reason that a lot of people go gluten-free to support their mental health. Research suggests that CD and non-celiac gluten sensitivity (NCGS) are linked to anxiety, depression, ADHD, and other mental health conditions. In fact, in one study, for every person with CD who had gut symptoms, eight had no digestive complaints at all.[2] Another study on NCGS found that the most common symptoms were fatigue, lack of well-being, headaches, anxiety, and brain fog.[3] The mechanism is complex, but in celiac disease, gluten triggers an autoimmune reaction that damages the gut lining, leading to inflammation and oxidative stress that can extend to the brain. Malabsorption of key nutrients—such as B vitamins, magnesium, zinc, and iron—can further harm neurotransmitter production, contributing to mood disorders. Even in NCGS, gluten-related inflammation may play a role in cognitive and emotional symptoms.

However, gluten-free diets can also carry risks. One study found that people without celiac disease who followed a gluten-free diet had lower levels of beneficial gut bacteria and less production of short-chain fatty acids, both of which support gut health and immune function.[4] While going gluten-free may relieve certain symptoms, it can also create nutritional gaps that could impact long-term health.

If I thought a gluten-free diet might be worth trying with a client, we'd take it slow. Instead of eliminating gluten immediately, we would establish a baseline through lab tests, including fasting glucose and hemoglobin A1c to assess blood sugar regulation as many gluten-free foods such as breads and crackers are higher on the glycemic index than their wheat-based counterparts. I'd also analyze their current diet to identify potential nutrient gaps—particularly in fiber, B vitamins, vitamin D, iron, calcium, magnesium, selenium, and zinc. If their current diet is already low in these critical nutrients, I can assume that a gluten-free diet would be increasingly nutritionally challenging. If, after weighing the risks and benefits, we decided to proceed, we would create a plan to replace lost nutrients, maintain gut health, and monitor any changes in energy, digestion, and mental well-being.

When it comes to making any major dietary change, it's critical to weigh both the potential nutrition benefits and the risks. If a dietary adjustment truly supports your health, it's worth doing in a thoughtful, balanced way. And if you're unsure? That's where working with a nutrition provider who understands both the benefits and potential risk of dietary changes can help you navigate adjustments that truly improve your well-being rather than inadvertently compromising it.

Is This Change Realistically Accessible to Me in Terms of Flexibility, Cost, and Availability?

It's easy to get caught up in the idea of an ideal diet—the perfectly curated meal plan that promises better energy, clearer skin, or a happier gut. But before making any major changes, it's essential to ask, "Is this even practical for my life?"

The best dietary approach isn't just the one that looks good on paper or sounds appealing in theory—it's the one you can actually sustain. That means considering not just the nutritional and health benefits, but also the logistics:

- Can I afford this way of eating?
- Are the foods I need available at my local grocery store?
- Will I have the time and ability to prepare meals this way?
- Does this diet fit into my life, or does my life have to revolve around it?

Can You Actually Get the Food?

Let's start with the basics: Can you reliably access the foods this diet requires?

There's a huge difference between a diet that's theoretically possible and one that's realistically accessible based on where you live. If a dietary change means constantly hunting down specialty ingredients, making long drives to health food stores, or paying for expensive subscription services, that's not sustainable for most people.

The Privilege of Eating Unprocessed Foods

Eating a whole-food, minimally processed diet sounds great in theory, but in practice, it often comes with enormous time, financial, and resource demands.

When my son was diagnosed with eosinophilic esophagitis, a chronic condition that causes difficulty swallowing due to inflammation in the esophagus, his allergist, gastroenterologist, and pediatrician all agreed a major elimination diet was needed to avoid triggers. We eliminated wheat, dairy, soy, eggs, tree nuts, peanuts, rice, corn, mustard, beef, and lentils.

Overnight, our world changed. Bread? We had to make it from scratch. Crackers? Yep, those too. Barbecue sauce? Only if we bought a dozen separate ingredients and made it ourselves. It felt like we had been transported back to the 1800s—there was no "grab and go." Every meal required planning, time, and considerable energy. I cooked three meals a day, seven days a week, for years.

Two things became very clear:

- Eating unprocessed food is time-consuming.
- Eating unprocessed food can be expensive.

This experience opened my eyes to how much privilege is embedded in wellness advice that glorifies homemade, "from-scratch" eating. It assumes you have access to specialty ingredients, the money to afford them, and the time, energy, and health to prepare everything yourself. Not everyone has that flexibility.

When we talk about healthy eating, we have to hold two truths at once. Yes, research is increasingly showing that diets high in ultra-processed foods are potentially problematic. Eating more whole foods can absolutely support your nervous system and long-term health. At the same time, we have to acknowledge that eating a completely unprocessed diet isn't always accessible, affordable, or sustainable.

That's why the most supportive nutrition approach is one rooted in both science and self-compassion. Sometimes, the most nourishing choice is the one that simply gets you fed. "Fed is best" isn't just a saying—it's a survival truth. You don't need to eat perfectly to care for your body; you just need to eat in ways that are doable, kind, and gently supportive of your current capacity.

For example, someone in a major city with access to large grocery stores and farmers' markets might have no problem following a diet that emphasizes fresh produce and niche health foods. But if you live in a rural area or rely on budget-friendly supermarkets, a diet that requires obscure ingredients might not be an option.

The same goes for seasonality. If a diet heavily relies on fresh berries, tropical fruits, or specific leafy greens, what happens when they're out of season? Will frozen versions work? Can you swap ingredients without compromising nutritional balance?

Does This Fit Your Budget?

Food trends often lean toward expensive options—grass-fed meats, wild-caught fish, organic everything, and superfoods that can double as mortgage payments. While nutrition is important, affordability matters too.

If a diet requires you to spend double or triple your current grocery budget just to follow it, it's probably not a sustainable option. And if sticking to it causes intense stress over finances, that stress can cancel out many of the potential health benefits.

Some things to ask yourself:

- Is this way of eating more expensive than what I currently do?
- Are there more affordable alternatives that provide the same nutritional benefit? (Example: lentils instead of organic quinoa, frozen veggies instead of fresh.)
- Will this change require costly specialty items or supplements?
- Am I willing (and able) to prioritize spending on this diet long-term?

The best diet for you is one that supports your health without putting financial strain on other areas of your life.

Is This Way of Eating True to You?

It's easy to fall into the trap of thinking that if you just eat like that influencer, wellness blogger, or friend who "figured it out," you'll look like them, feel like them, or live like them. Social media is flooded with "What I Eat in a Day" videos, perfectly curated grocery hauls and morning routines that suggest there's a formula for feeling good in your body. But here's the truth: Your most nourishing way of eating won't come from copying someone else. It has to come from you.

When we choose a diet because we hope it will make us look or feel like someone else, we disconnect from what our body is asking for. We start outsourcing our inner wisdom to external rules, images, and identities that don't actually fit who we are. It's a subtle but powerful way of abandoning ourselves.

A sustainable way of eating that truly supports you should feel like it brings you home to yourself—not like you're fighting your body, your identity, or your needs to fit someone else's template.

When a diet aligns with your needs, it tends to feel grounding and supportive. It increases your capacity to show up for your life, not just physically but emotionally and socially. You feel more like yourself and are able to engage with the world.

When a diet is not aligned, it often feels like pressure. You might find yourself obsessing over what's allowed, hyperfocused on tracking and measuring, avoiding social situations or feeling disconnected from your own body signals. You may notice that instead of feeling better you feel smaller emotionally. Less joy. Less energy. Less freedom.

Before adopting someone else's nutrition advice, ask yourself:

- Am I choosing this because it genuinely feels supportive, or because I hope it will make me more like someone else?
- Does this way of eating help me feel connected to myself—my body, my needs, my rhythms?
- Does this bring me a sense of ease and ventral regulation, or a sense of tension or pressure?

Food should be a tool for supporting the life you want, not something that becomes the center of your life or a measure of your worth.

Final Thoughts: If It's Not Accessible, It's Not Sustainable

A diet that doesn't fit into your real life isn't a diet that will last. Before committing to a change, take the time to consider the logistics, the costs, and the flexibility. If it works only in perfect conditions, it's not actually working.

A dietary shift that enhances health should feel sustainable, adaptable, and aligned with your real-life circumstances, not just a theoretical ideal. If an approach is too costly, time-consuming, stressful, or impractical, it's unlikely to be beneficial in the long run.

True nourishment comes from choices that are both evidence-based and personally accessible, allowing you to maintain well-being without unnecessary strain. The most effective diet is the one that works *for you*, not the one that looks good on paper or fits someone else's idea of "healthy."

PART II
What Comes After Your Body Keeps the Score?

Trauma doesn't just live in our memories—it leaves fingerprints all over the body. Bessel van der Kolk's book *The Body Keeps the Score* helped many people first understand this: trauma reshapes our nervous system, shifts our digestion and metabolism, and can even set the stage for chronic health conditions. When the body stays stuck in survival mode for too long, it's not just your mood that takes a hit—it's everything from your immune system to your blood sugar to your gut health.

In my work with clients, I use a simple structure to help make sense of these changes. It's called the **FIGS protocol**, and it looks at four areas that often get disrupted by trauma: **food, inflammation, gut, and stress**. When someone comes to me with a trauma history or mental health symptoms, we don't just ask, "What's wrong?"—we ask, "What needs support?"

- Does your food give your brain and body the fuel they need?
- Is there inflammation quietly stirring up fatigue or pain?
- Can your gut digest and absorb what you're giving it?
- And how is your nervous system handling the daily load of stress?

This section of the book is about how trauma shows up physically —and how, gently, we can start to meet the body's needs with more care and less judgment. But let's set one thing straight before we dive in: This isn't another self-improvement project.

I'm not here to add twenty new things to your to-do list or to make you feel like you're failing if you don't start meditating, drinking green smoothies, or buying every supplement at the health food store.

As KC Davis reminds us in *How to Keep House While Drowning*, care tasks are morally neutral—even when they're health related.

You are not a bad person if you miss a workout, if cooking dinner feels overwhelming, or if your vitamin bottle gathers dust on the shelf (I'm right there with you!). You are still good. Still worthy. Still whole.

Think of this section as a menu, not a mandate. These ideas aren't here to pressure you—they're here to meet you where you are. From a regulated state, you may find you have more energy and curiosity to try a new approach. And if you don't right now, that's okay too. Healing doesn't come from perfect behavior—it comes from choice, and from tiny moments of self-kindness.

You'll also notice that I've deliberately kept things simple. Too much information can overwhelm an already taxed nervous system. Instead of giving you a hundred possible ideas, I'll offer just a handful for each topic—enough to give you options, but not so many that you get stuck in decision fatigue. Take what serves you. Leave the rest. You can always come back later.

CHAPTER 5

FIGS Starts with Food: Are You Getting What You Need?

Having a healthy relationship with food means you are not morally superior or inferior based on your eating choices.

–Evelyn Tribole, *Intuitive Eating: A Revolutionary Program That Works*

Singer James Blunt, best known for his hit song "You're Beautiful," gave himself scurvy in college after deciding to eat nothing but meat and mayonnaise for two months. He developed severe fatigue, joint pain, and other classic symptoms of vitamin C deficiency—something most of us assume only happened to sailors in the 1700s.[1] While Blunt's extreme diet may sound ridiculous, it highlights an important truth: nutrient deficiencies still exist today. While full-blown deficiencies are less common, subclinical insufficiencies—nutrient levels that aren't low enough to cause an immediate medical crisis but still fall short of supporting optimal health—are far more common. A study published in *The Lancet* found that more than 5 billion people worldwide do not consume enough iodine, vitamin E, and calcium, while more than 4 billion people lack sufficient iron, riboflavin, folate, and vitamin C.[2] In the United States, nearly half the population isn't getting enough vitamin A or C, and the numbers are even higher for vitamin D and E—95 percent and 84 percent, respectively. Even zinc falls short for about 15 percent of people.[3]

This chapter begins the first step of the FIGS protocol: food—examining the nutrients that can play a role in mental health, trauma-related symptoms, and conditions commonly developed after trauma. Unlike severe deficiencies including scurvy or rickets, insufficiencies may not lead to dramatic symptoms, but over time, they can quietly wear down resilience, impact mood, energy levels, and the body's ability to handle stress.

Cooking Up Regulation: How Food Helps Shape Mental Health

Imagine for a moment that supporting your mental health was like cooking a meal. I know, I know, this is a hard stretch coming from a nutritionist. Humor me, though.

You'll need to get the raw ingredients, read the instructions, apply the right techniques and temperature, and eventually—barring a disaster on the stove—you'll have a yummy dish. In the same way, your body relies on bioactive compounds from food—vitamins, minerals, amino acids, fats, and polyphenols—as the raw ingredients it needs to "cook up" mental health. These nutrients are more than fuel; they are information and building blocks. Once inside the body, they're transformed through biochemical processes into the neurotransmitters, hormones, and cellular signals that support mood, focus, sleep, and emotional resilience. What you eat quite literally becomes part of how you feel.

Before you go to a place of shame and blame that you aren't eating "right" and that's why you feel so anxious or depressed, let me stop you. Sure, you may be one of those people that just doesn't eat enough protein, and eating more protein makes you feel like a rock star. But you also may be someone who eats well most of the time, consuming well-balanced meals on the regular. If this sounds more like you, remember that a delicious meal isn't just the sum of the ingredients used to create it; it also requires significant preparation and monitoring.

In short, you can eat all the right things, and the nervous system "oven" with which you're trying to cook up supportive mental health is either stuck on high (sympathetic activation) or running really low (dorsal shutdown). If you're really unlucky, that nervous system oven is switching on and off unpredictably, throwing an extra dose of chaos into the recipe (it's both burnt and raw!). Ventral regulation allows your body to take the ingredients you've provided it and bake them into a delicious dish—emotional and physical well-being.

That's why, as we start to talk about food, I'm going to remind you to watch your nervous system during this chapter, and if you feel yourself going into a survival state, either take a break and walk away for a while, or even go to the next chapter and see if that feels more accessible.

You might notice I'm not asking you to follow a specific dietary pattern here. I'm not telling you to "try keto," "go gluten-free," or "eat a Mediterranean diet"—and that's entirely intentional. In my experience, sweeping nutrition overhauls often feel overwhelming, especially when someone is already navigating stress or dysregulation.

Even something labeled as "simple"—such as the Mediterranean diet—isn't actually simple when you look at what it asks of you in terms of planning, ingredients, and consistency. That kind of all-in change can feel like a stressor, not a support. Instead, I'd rather have you start with small, doable shifts—such as adding more protein to breakfast or including a mineral-rich snack. We'll still touch on the research around different dietary patterns and mental health in the sidebars, but here in the main text, we're going to keep it grounded in what feels realistic for your nervous system today.

Eat Well-Balanced Meals

Well-balanced meals are incredibly unsexy. Why? They lack the drama of an extreme approach, and they get fewer social media likes than an extreme food elimination diet. In the age of *nutritionism*—a term popularized by Michael Pollan to describe the focus on individual nutrients rather than whole foods—the well-balanced meal has lost its spotlight. We hear "cut the carbs, find your clarity" and "detox your plate, detox your life" much more often than "eat nutritionally complete meals."

So why does it matter? Because health isn't built on hype. A well-balanced meal may not go viral, but it nourishes the body in ways we don't fully understand yet. When we eat whole, varied meals, we get the known nutrients—and the still-undiscovered ones that quietly support our mental, metabolic, and emotional health.

Does When You Eat Affect How You Feel?

A large study of nearly 35,000 adults in the United States explored not just *what* people eat, but *when* they eat—and how it might affect depression symptoms.[4]

Researchers found that people who consumed a higher percentage of their calories from snacks and nonmeal times tended to report more depressive symptoms. On the other hand, those who ate a bigger portion of their daily calories at breakfast—especially if breakfast made up at least 20 percent of their total intake—reported fewer symptoms of depression.

In short, when it comes to mood, *when* you eat might matter almost as much as *what* you eat.

A well-balanced plate doesn't require you to calculate macros or track every bite. There are many ways to nourish the body—and what balance looks like depends on your traditions, preferences, access, and needs on any given day. Ask yourself what meals feel grounding and energizing to you. What does a satisfying and complete meal look like in your family, your community, or your culture? How does your meal support steadiness, connection, or healing?

What's the Deal with the Mediterranean Diet?

You've probably heard about the Mediterranean diet before—maybe from your doctor, a magazine article, or that friend who suddenly bought a lot of olive oil. This dietary pattern reflects food traditions from a wide variety of countries that border the Mediterranean Sea—places such as Morocco, Greece, Italy, and Spain. While each of these cultures has a distinct culinary identity, they also have shared patterns such as cooking with olive oil, eating plenty of fresh fruit and vegetables, including legumes and fish, and centering meals around a community experience. This way of eating isn't just trendy—it's one of the best-researched dietary patterns for supporting overall health, including mental and nervous system health.

At its core, the Mediterranean diet emphasizes whole, unprocessed foods: lots of colorful plants, healthy fats (such as olive oil), fish, legumes, whole grains, and fermented dairy. What makes it especially interesting from a trauma-informed perspective is that it's been shown to influence the autonomic nervous system—the part of your body that controls stress responses. One study even compared the Mediterranean diet to a fast food-style diet and found that the Mediterranean approach was linked with more parasympathetic (i.e., calming) nervous system activity while fast food was linked with increased sympathetic (i.e., stress) activity.[5]

It gets better: Adaptations such as the *green* Mediterranean diet (with even more plant-based foods) have been shown to reduce systemic and neuroinflammation, improve immune regulation, and even support changes in gene expression that lower disease risk. Components such as fiber, omega-3s, and polyphenols (the antioxidants in fruits, veggies, herbs, and olive oil) help nourish the gut and brain, keeping those systems communicating smoothly.[6]

There's even research that shows this style of eating can help buffer the body's stress response by positively influencing the gut microbiome, supporting the intestinal barrier, and calming immune responses.[7] In other words, it's not just about preventing heart disease—this way of eating helps support resilience from the inside out.

That said, this is *not* a one-size-fits-all prescription. You don't need to fully switch your lifestyle or buy imported cheese to benefit. Even incorporating a few Mediterranean-inspired elements—such as adding olive oil, choosing legumes more often, or including fermented yogurt or greens—can support your nervous system and mood over time.

And it's not just about the food itself. You can also focus on the community aspects of eating that are central to Mediterranean cultures—things such as sharing a meal with others, slowing down while you eat, cooking with family or friends, or turning meals into a time of connection rather than rushing or multitasking. These practices are powerful for nervous system regulation, too, because nourishment isn't just what's on your plate; it's also the experience of being in ventral regulation while you eat.

Across the world, cultures have long practiced their own versions of balance—pairing foods that bring energy, satisfaction, and nourishment. While modern Western nutrition often breaks meals down into macronutrients, many traditional foodways offer balance through rhythm, variety, seasonality, and a deep relationship with the land.

Here are just a few examples:

- **Indigenous and First Nations tradition.** Meals with corn, beans, and squash. These foods grow together and support one another in the soil—just as they support energy, protein, and fiber in the body.

- **Ayurvedic tradition (South Asia).** Meals may include rice, dal, vegetables, yogurt, and pickles. This pattern combines all six tastes (sweet, salty, bitter, pungent, sour, astringent) and offers warm, grounding nourishment for digestion and dosha balance.

- **Mediterranean pattern.** Couscous, white fish, beans, vegetables, and olive oil. A pattern focused on variety, seasonal produce, and heart-healthy fats, often eaten communally and slowly.

- **Latin American tradition.** Plantains, beans, meat, and vegetables. Meals are often built around staples and variety, combining comfort, satiety, and cultural continuity.

- **Western nutrition framework.** Chicken breast, baked potato with butter, fresh vegetable salad with vinaigrette. Often framed around macronutrient categories: protein, starch, fat, fiber.

Balance doesn't have a universal recipe. It's about what works for you and your lifestyle.

For someone who loves to cook:

- **Think anchor plus variety.** Start with protein as this has grounding properties, then pair with vegetables, carbs, and condiments to make meals..

- **Batch cook base ingredients.** Grains, starches, and proteins can be made in advance and then mixed and matched throughout the week.

- **Explore dishes that naturally have all the components.** Try stir fries, bibimbap, tacos, curries, or smoothies that contain protein, fruit and vegetables, and fat.

For someone who buys pre-prepared meals:

- **Check the label for variety.** Does it include protein, carbs, and fiber (from veggies or whole grains)?

- **Add a side or a topping.** Pair a frozen entree with a bagged salad, precut fruit, or a microwaved veggie pouch.

- **Keep flexible add-ons on hand.** Buy hardboiled eggs, hummus, rotisserie chicken, Greek yogurt, canned beans, or nuts to round things out.

For someone who eats out regularly:

- **Scan the menu for what's missing.** Once you've chosen your meal, explore if adding a side of veggies, beans, or soup or salad would add nutritional balance.

- **Choose meals with mixed elements.** Burrito bowls, Thai

curries, or poke often include protein, carbs, and vegetables naturally.

- **Ask for small tweaks.** Request extra vegetables or see if you can swap the fries for half salad/half fries.

Balance is often about what you add, not what you take away. If there is a single experiment you choose out of this chapter, let it be to explore how eating regular, nutritionally complete meals make you feel. After all, balanced meals don't just feed your cells and give you the best chance to meet your nutrient needs; they also feed your sense of safety. The predictability of a full plate, the rhythm of regular meals, and the satisfaction of eating enough to satisfy and satiate can tell your nervous system you aren't in danger right now.

Fuel for Energy

A really common conversation I have with clients—and one that surprises people—is about eating more, not less. We tend to assume that if something feels "off" with our body, the solution must involve cutting something out. But in reality, many people simply aren't eating enough energy (calories) to fully support their needs, and when they start eating more, they feel dramatically better.

It makes sense—your body needs fuel to function. Without enough energy, your brain struggles to focus, your mood takes a hit, and your body prioritizes only the most essential functions, leaving you feeling sluggish, cold, irritable, and exhausted. Over time, chronically low energy intake can contribute to hormone imbalances, gut issues, poor sleep, and increased stress sensitivity—all of which can make it even harder to function day-to-day.

Some people intentionally eat less because of diet culture messaging, but many people don't realize they're under-eating until they take a closer look. Maybe you're skipping meals because you're busy, drinking coffee instead of eating breakfast, or just not feeling hungry due to stress. Maybe you're eating foods that don't keep you full, leading to a pattern of low intake early in the day followed by extreme hunger (and sometimes overeating) at night. Whatever the reason, if you're running on too little fuel, your body will eventually push back.

Signs You Might Not Be Eating Enough Energy:

- Mental health symptoms: Brain fog, difficulty concentrating, irritability, anxiety, low mood, or a sense of emotional numbness
- Physical symptoms: Fatigue, dizziness, feeling cold, frequent headaches, trouble sleeping, hair thinning, hormone imbalances, or digestive issues such as bloating and constipation
- Patterns that suggest low intake: Skipping meals, relying heavily on caffeine to get through the day, feeling ravenous at night, or frequently feeling "too full" after small portions

If any of this sounds familiar, try experimenting with eating more and see how you feel. This doesn't mean forcing yourself to eat if you're not hungry but rather checking in on your patterns and adding more food consistently throughout the day—especially earlier in the day. Some of my clients start with something simple, such as making sure they have a balanced breakfast or adding a snack in the afternoon, and they notice big improvements in mood, energy, and focus within just a few days.

Your body needs fuel, and getting enough energy isn't about overeating—it's about giving your brain, nervous system, and entire body what they need to function optimally. If you suspect you've been running on too little, try adding more and see what happens.

Choose Sources of Protein

In many ways, amino acids are the building blocks of mood. Found within protein-rich foods such as meat, fish, tofu, beans, lentils, and nuts, amino acids are broken down in the gut and turned into handy chemicals such as serotonin, dopamine, and GABA—all crucial for mental health and gut-brain communication.

Without adequate protein, the gut and brain can't produce the neurotransmitters needed in the gut to be able to send messages of safety to the brain. Serotonin produced in the gut can indirectly influence mood and mental health through the gut-brain axis, even though it doesn't cross the blood-brain barrier directly. Instead, it communicates with the brain through the vagus nerve and through modulating the gut immune system to reduce inflammation. While brain-derived serotonin is crucial for regulating mood, sleep, and appetite, gut serotonin contributes to mental well-being by ensuring that the gut remains balanced, comfortable, and responsive. The gut's serotonin helps maintain a stable environment, which can help reduce stressful gut feelings that might send the brain into overdrive.

If you eat too little protein, and therefore have fewer amino acids available to make serotonin or dopamine, you might have a problem. Over the years, there have been a number of acute tryptophan depletion studies, where researchers reduce or eliminate people's intake of tryptophan, and watch their mood. With the removal of tryptophan, and therefore the potential for less serotonin synthesis, some study participants get depressed and anxious. To be clear, adding protein isn't a miracle cure for everyone's mood issues, especially if you're already eating plenty of protein. But I always think that getting a little extra protein is a great place to start experimenting.

Protein is having a moment these days. Between the protein-powder-chugging gym bro warriors to the addition of cottage cheese to nearly every recipe you see on social media, protein is winning the battle for public awareness—and for good reason. Not only is protein needed by the body to make neurotransmitters, the amino acids contained in it are also a preferred fuel source for the gut, which, as we'll discuss in future chapters, is essential for mental health.

Protein Does More Than You Think

Protein isn't just for building muscle; it plays a crucial role in nearly every system of the body. It supports the nervous, immune, metabolic, and hormonal systems, helping to keep everything in balance. There are many factors that can impact your protein needs, including your age, the amount of physical and psychological stress you experience, and your health status. Your body relies on protein to produce antibodies that fight off illness, hemoglobin to carry oxygen in the blood, and hormones such as thyroid hormone and insulin. It's also essential for making neurotransmitters–the brain chemicals that influence mood, focus, and emotional regulation. Getting enough protein each day helps your body stay strong, steady, and resilient.

If you're not sure whether you're getting enough protein, try experimenting for a few days. Add a little more to each meal and notice how you feel—more steady, more clearheaded, less snacky or foggy? It doesn't need to be a dramatic overhaul. Sometimes, a few extra spoonfuls of lentils or an extra egg can make a surprising difference. Eggs, beans, yogurt, peanut butter, tofu, chicken—all of these are basic, accessible sources of protein you can add.

Don't Fear Fats

Throughout the 1980s and 1990s, foods high in fat needed a decent publicist. The evening news, talk shows, and even professional organizations such as the American Cardiology Association decried

fat sources including eggs, thinking that it would push up our cholesterol. Frankenfoods, such as the fat substitute Olestra, popped up
with the goal to add no fat or calories to fried foods. Unfortunately,
Olestra also caused rampant diarrhea and is now rarely seen in food
products.

Thankfully, multiple meta-analyses and large-scale studies
have proven that fat isn't the enemy, and in fact, it is essential for
mental health—if you want to think clearly and feel steady, fat isn't
optional.[8,9,10]

What About Keto?

The ketogenic diet—often called *keto*—has gotten a lot of
attention for its potential mental health benefits. And while
it's definitely not the right fit for everyone, there's growing evidence that it may help reduce inflammation in the brain and improve how the nervous system functions for certain individuals.

At its core, keto is a high-fat, very low-carbohydrate way of
eating that shifts your body into a state called *ketosis*. This metabolic change allows your body to burn fat for energy instead
of carbohydrates. For some people, this shift can support brain
function, reduce neuroinflammation, and even reshape the gut
microbiome in helpful ways.[11]

In fact, keto has been shown to influence the gut-brain
connection in multiple ways. It can impact the HPA axis (your
central stress response system), reduce gut permeability, calm
inflammation, and stimulate the vagus nerve—helping improve
digestion, mood, and resilience to stress. It may also change
how genes are expressed in the brain, especially in areas such
as the prefrontal cortex and amygdala that affect focus, fear,
and decision-making.[12]

Keto also seems to reduce stress-related inflammation and
support the production and balance of key brain chemicals

such as glutamate and GABA. It even enhances mitochondrial function and antioxidant activity in the brain, which can protect against cellular stress over time.[13]

A big note of caution here: I do *not* recommend trying a ketogenic diet without support from a knowledgeable, trauma-informed nutrition provider. While keto can help some people, it can also feel highly restrictive, triggering, or dysregulating–especially if you have a history of trauma, disordered eating, or rigid food rules. Your body and your story matter. There's no one-size-fits-all approach, and this isn't something to jump into lightly.

If you're curious, bring it into a conversation with a Certified Nutrition Specialist (CNS) or Registered Dietitian (RD) that you trust–one who can help you experiment gently, safely, and with your whole self in mind.

One form of fat I particularly emphasize with clients is omega-3s. In the decade I've been working as a licensed nutritionist, I've seen plenty of normal omega-3 index results—but almost exclusively in people who supplement. Among those who don't take omega-3 supplements, I've only seen three labs come back in the optimal range. Three. In ten years. Of those three normal results, two belonged to my nutrition interns—who already knew how to optimize their diet for omega-3s—so I don't really think they count.

The omega-3 index, which measures the percentage of eicosapentaenoic acid (EPA) and docosahexaenoic acid (DHA) in red blood cell membranes, is often a reliable marker of long-term omega-3 status, with levels above 8 percent considered optimal and levels below 4 percent indicating significant deficiency.[14] These essential fats have potent anti-inflammatory properties, which can help mitigate inflammation, a factor that is often linked to mood disorders. Research suggests that higher intakes of omega-3s are associated with a reduced risk of depression and anxiety.

If you want to add more omega-3s to your diet, here are a few ways my clients have used:

- **Seaweed and algae.** Crumble over rice, noodles, or avocado toast.
- **Canned salmon.** I often make salmon cakes using canned salmon (it's cheaper!) with an egg and some breadcrumbs.
- **Flaxseed oil.** Try it in salad dressings or drizzled on soups.
- **Ground flaxseeds.** Add them to your cereal or try in salads or smoothies.
- **Purslane.** Use it fresh in salads or sauté with eggs and greens.
- **Chia seeds.** Use them in your overnight oats or morning smoothie.
- **Walnuts.** Make a walnut-heavy trail mix for snacking.

You can also add an omega-3 supplement if eating omegas on a regular basis is challenging. Watch out for brands that have a large total dose of fish oil (in this case, 1,000 mg) but a small amount of the types of omegas that we really want for mental health (EPA and DHA). As you can see below, the dose in both supplements is the same: 1,000 mg. However, the supplement to the right has a substantially higher amount of omega-3s, with 95 percent of the total content of the capsule to be EPA and DHA, versus 34 percent of the capsule to the left. Aim for a total quantity of fish oil to be 1,000 to 2,000 mg (one to two grams), with the vast majority being EPA and DHA.

**Different Brands,
Different Amounts
of Omegas**
(No, this is NOT standardized . . .)

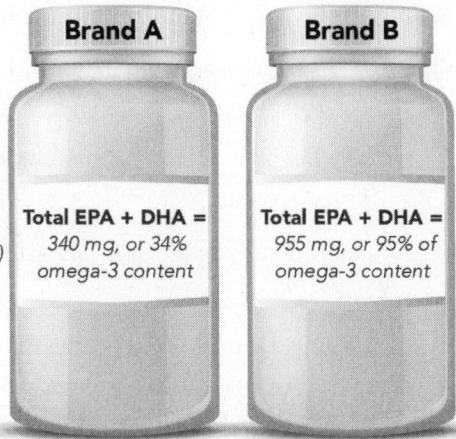

Brand A

Total EPA + DHA =
*340 mg, or 34%
omega-3 content*

Brand B

Total EPA + DHA =
*955 mg, or 95% of
omega-3 content*

Less Omega   **More Omega**

Same Price

Not all omega-3 supplements are created equal. These two bottles contain the
same amount of total fish oil, but only one delivers a high dose of EPA and DHA.

Even if your diet is well-balanced, nutrient availability isn't *just*
about what you eat—it's also about what's in the food itself. Modern
farming practices have significantly depleted soil nutrients, meaning
that today's vegetables contain 20 to 80 percent less vitamins and
minerals than they did just a few generations ago. For example, iron
levels in vegetables such as onions, watercress, and collard greens
have dropped by more than 50 percent, and fruits such as bananas
and strawberries have lost more than half their iron and vitamin A
content.[15]

Dietary restrictions can also play a role in nutrient insufficiencies. Vegan and vegetarian diets may be low in B12 and iron, while
low-fat diets can reduce the intake of fat-soluble vitamins such as A,
D, E, and K. People on low-carb diets may struggle to get enough
fiber, magnesium, potassium, and vitamins A, C, D, and E.[16] And
even gluten-free diets can be problematic. Often, gluten-free diets
lack fiber, and vitamins D, B12, and folate, as well as minerals such
asiron, zinc, magnesium, and calcium.[17]

What About Going Gluten-Free?

You've probably heard a lot about gluten-free diets—and not just for people with celiac disease. While going gluten-free is essential for anyone with celiac, some people without the disease may also benefit from cutting back on gluten-containing foods. This is sometimes called *nonceliac gluten sensitivity* (NCGS).

For individuals who have this sensitivity, gluten can trigger low-grade inflammation in the gut, increasing something called *intestinal permeability*. You might hear this referred to as "leaky gut." When the gut barrier becomes more porous, it allows unwanted substances such as toxins and inflammatory compounds into the bloodstream—and from there, they can affect the brain and nervous system.

Emerging research suggests this might also impact the *blood-brain barrier*, the protective shield that usually keeps harmful substances out of the brain. When this barrier becomes more permeable, it may open the door to inflammation in the central nervous system, contributing to symptoms such as anxiety, depression, or brain fog.[18]

A gluten-free diet isn't automatically healthier, and it's not necessary—or even helpful—for everyone. If you notice gut issues, brain fog, or mood shifts after eating gluten-containing foods, it's worth getting curious but not restrictive. Sometimes, the issue isn't gluten itself, but something else in the food. For example, many wheat-based foods are high in FODMAPs, a group of fermentable carbohydrates that can trigger bloating, gas, or discomfort in people with sensitive digestion.

That's why I don't recommend eliminating gluten on your own. Instead, work with a knowledgeable, trauma-informed CNS or RD who can help you explore your symptoms through thoughtful food experiments. That way, you can avoid unnecessary restrictions and better understand what your body truly needs.

Medications can further interfere with absorption—as an example, the use of the immunosuppressant drug methotrexate, commonly prescribed for rheumatoid arthritis, can inhibit folate's conversion into the active form of the vitamin, leading to symptoms that are alleviated by taking folate.[19] And then there's gut health; conditions such as IBS, Crohn's disease, or even chronic stress can harm nutrient absorption, making it difficult for the body to access essential vitamins and minerals.

At the same time, overconsumption of certain nutrients can be a real concern. Many people assume that if a little is good, more must be better—but some vitamins and minerals have an established Tolerable Upper Intake Level (UL), meaning excessive amounts can lead to unpleasant or even harmful effects. I learned this firsthand with magnesium.

I always sleep better when I add a little magnesium to my nightly tea—it helps me unwind. But one night, just as I was scooping the powder into my cup, I got distracted and walked away. When I came back, I couldn't remember if I'd already added my magnesium. Erring on the side of relaxation, I tossed in another big, heaping scoop for good measure and settled onto the couch with my tea. Not long after, my body made it abundantly clear that I had hit bowel tolerance for magnesium, leading to a series of urgent, unfortunate trips to the bathroom. Lesson learned: Super-sizing vitamins and minerals doesn't always lead to great results.

When addressing nutrient needs with clients, I take a comprehensive approach rather than focusing on just one nutrient. I begin by analyzing the diet, identifying patterns, and looking for key vitamin and mineral gaps. From there, I work to fill those gaps using food-based strategies and, when necessary, supplementation.

What I won't do is spend months trying to correct a single deficiency—such as low vitamin D—while assuming it alone will resolve mental health symptoms. If a nutrient is low, I'll absolutely address it, but at the same time, I'll support other critical nutrition and lifestyle factors that influence mental well-being. This includes improving overall dietary quality, stabilizing blood sugar, supporting gut health, and ensuring adequate intake of other key nutrients such as magnesium, omega-3s, and B vitamins.

Mental health and nutrition are both complex, and real progress comes from a holistic, evidence-based approach—not quick fixes. With that in mind, the rest of this chapter will outline the key nutritional targets I assess and address with every client experiencing mental health symptoms.

For each of these targets, I'll encourage you to ask yourself a guiding question: Am I currently getting enough? And if not, how could I add more? This approach helps shift the focus from rigid rules or overwhelming lists of recommendations to something much more practical: identifying where your intake may be low and what small, meaningful steps you can take to increase it. By tuning into these questions, you can start making adjustments that support both your body and mind in a sustainable way.

Before we dive in, I want to offer a word of caution. It's easy to feel overwhelmed when reading about multiple nutritional factors— some people may respond by ordering fifteen different supplements, while others feel so paralyzed that they shut the book and walk away. I don't wish either extreme for you. Intentionally look for something to do that is a stretch, not a stress. Stretch means possible within ventral regulation; stress means a visit to a survival state.

Watch Your Vitamin D Levels

I keep an eye on vitamin D levels in my practice, and without supplementation, I've only seen *forty-five normal results* in my entire career. Granted, I live and work in Illinois, where the sun isn't exactly generous year-round, and the people who seek my help often have health concerns that predispose them to lower levels. But still. About 35 percent of adults in the United States have a vitamin D deficiency, and up to 1 billion people worldwide have subclinical vitamin D deficiency—meaning their levels are low enough to cause concern, even if they don't meet the threshold for a true deficiency.[20] If you have a mental health diagnosis, your levels might be worth checking. While extreme deficiencies can lead to rickets or osteomalacia, even moderate insufficiencies have been linked to anxiety and depression as well as muscle weakness, gum disease, and even bone pain.[21]

Vitamin D is often called the "sunshine vitamin" because your body can produce it when your skin is exposed to sunlight. Specifically, ultraviolet B (UVB) rays trigger a process in the skin that converts cholesterol into vitamin D. However, this process is influenced by multiple factors, including the time of year, latitude, skin pigmentation, age, and sunscreen use, as well as air pollution, the gut microbiome, and the health of your liver and kidneys.

The National Institutes of Health recommends five to thirty minutes of sun exposure to the face, arms, hands, and legs twice a week, particularly between 10 AM and 3 PM[22] In contrast, the American Academy of Dermatology advises against intentional sun exposure for vitamin D synthesis due to the risk of skin cancer. Instead, they recommend getting adequate vitamin D through diet and supplements.[23]

This is where it gets tricky. While vitamin D production is the most well-established benefit of sun exposure, emerging research suggests that sunlight may have additional benefits beyond vitamin D, including effects on the immune system, mood, sleep, and circadian rhythms. At the same time, it's clear that UV exposure also carries risks.

That's why I always emphasize that my clients should talk to a primary care provider or a dermatologist to help them assess personal skin cancer risk and determine an approach to sun exposure that balances risks and benefits.

Regardless of which guideline you choose to follow, if you live in a northern climate, UVB rays are too weak during the winter months to produce sufficient vitamin D, meaning many people become deficient unless they supplement or get enough from food.

In addition to helping your skin make vitamin D, sun exposure unfortunately also increases your risk of sunburn and oxidative damage. But your diet might offer a clever line of defense. Carotenoids—the colorful pigments found in foods such as carrots, sweet potatoes, tomatoes, and leafy greens—have been shown to enhance the skin's natural resistance to sunburn and other types of UV damage. I think of these foods as inside-out sun care—delicious and protective.[24]

Globally, human populations meet their vitamin D needs through seasonal food practices that prioritize nutrient-dense ingredients. In coastal and northern regions, people consume oily fish, organ meats, and animal fats—especially from animals exposed to sunlight—providing rich sources of vitamin D. Fermentation, drying, and preserving techniques not only extend the shelf life of these foods (hey there, pickled herring!) but also preserve their vitamin content through long winters or periods of scarcity. Many cultures regularly ate foods such as fish liver, blubber, eggs, sun-dried fish, and full-fat dairy from pasture-raised animals, all of which naturally contain vitamin D.[25]

If you want to add more vitamin D to your diet, here are a few options my clients have found helpful:

- **Cod liver oil.** Add a spoonful to a smoothie if you can handle the taste.
- **Egg yolks.** Include them in your breakfast and ditch the egg-white-only trend.
- **Oysters, clams, shrimp, and mussels.** Make cioppino, a traditional seafood stew.
- **Fortified plant-based milk.** Choose soy or almond milk if you don't consume dairy.
- **Canned tuna.** Snack on it for a convenient, shelf-stable source of vitamin D.

If you're a fan of mushrooms, you can also give them a sunbath to increase their vitamin D levels. Mushrooms naturally contain ergosterol, a compound that transforms into vitamin D2 when exposed to UV light—so giving them a sunbath, especially gill-side up, can significantly boost their vitamin D content. Just thirty to sixty minutes of sunlight can raise their vitamin D2 levels to meet or even exceed the daily recommended intake.[26]

Unlike some other nutrients, vitamin D can be tricky to get from food alone, especially if you don't eat a lot of the foods listed above.

If your last physical showed low vitamin D levels and you don't feel like you can devote time or effort to eating more vitamin D–rich foods or spending extra time outside, you're not alone. Many people rely on supplements, especially during the winter months or in places where sunlight is limited. If hitting your vitamin D needs through food feels impossible, supplementation can be a practical solution—but keep an eye on dosage. Most experts agree that 1,000 IU of vitamin D3 is an adequate dose if you don't get exposure to sunlight. More isn't always better, and excessive vitamin D intake can lead to toxicity over time. If you're supplementing, it's always a good idea to check with your healthcare provider to find the right balance for your needs.

Add Magnesium for Calm

If there's one simple step that can make a difference in anxiety and sleep, adding magnesium is it. Magnesium is a powerhouse mineral that helps regulate stress by balancing cortisol, your body's primary stress hormone. When levels are low, anxiety can spike, and sleep can suffer—creating a vicious cycle where stress worsens sleep, and poor sleep amplifies stress. Ensuring adequate magnesium intake can help break this cycle, promoting relaxation, better sleep, and a more resilient nervous system.

Low magnesium levels can contribute to increased anxiety, poor stress tolerance, and difficulty sleeping, making it harder for the nervous system to stay regulated.[27] Physically, signs of deficiency may include brittle or weak nails that split easily, frequent muscle twitching, and muscle cramps, all of which indicate that the body may not have enough magnesium to support optimal function.[28]

Traditionally, diets met magnesium needs through the regular consumption of whole, minimally processed plant foods such as legumes, leafy greens, seeds, nuts, bananas, and whole grains. These foods were often soaked, sprouted, or fermented to enhance absorption. Seaweed, a key part of coastal diets, provided magnesium, and bone broths made from whole animals, as well as small fish eaten with bones, contributed to the mineral intake as well.

If you want to add more magnesium-rich foods to your diet today, here are some easy ways:

- **Leafy greens.** My favorite is sautéed beet greens with garlic, but spinach and kale work just as well. Keep in mind that greens shrink a lot when cooked—raw greens take up a lot of fridge space, so you may prefer to buy them frozen.
- **Seed crackers.** Make or buy crackers that include pumpkin and chia seeds for a crunchy, magnesium-rich snack.
- **Teff and millet.** Use teff to make injera or add to porridge, and choose millet when you'd normally cook rice.
- **Taro.** Boil, steam, roast, and use like potatoes in soups and stews.
- **Almonds and cashews.** These nuts provide an easy, portable magnesium boost.
- **Black beans or pigeon peas.** Incorporate them into meals like soups, salads, or grain bowls—one cup of cooked black beans provides a good amount of magnesium.

Although there's a lot of hype about the different forms of supplemental magnesium, I generally stick to magnesium glycinate unless constipation is a concern, in which case I opt for magnesium citrate. While magnesium threonate is often marketed for its ability to cross the blood-brain barrier, the evidence that it is actually better than other, cheaper forms of supplemental magnesium is limited. Magnesium glycinate is well absorbed and gentle on the stomach, making it a practical choice for most people who want to supplement.

B Vitamins Support Energy

Recently, I had a client come back from their doctor and tell me their B vitamins were low. I asked which ones, and they didn't know. There are a bunch of B vitamins, and all of them have different jobs, so it is important to know which B vitamin we're talking about here.

B vitamins in general are essential for mental and physical health, playing a key role in energy production, neurotransmitter function, and red blood cell formation. Deficiencies in B12, folate, or B6 can contribute to mood imbalances, fatigue, and even neurological symptoms. Since B vitamins work together, if one is low, others may be as well, which is why I typically recommend a B complex rather than supplementing with individual B vitamins. Ideally, your diet provides enough of these crucial nutrients, but for those with absorption issues, restricted diets, or increased needs, targeted supplementation can help.

Traditionally, our diets emphasized the consumption of B vitamins through a wide variety of nutrient-dense, whole foods. Organ meats such as liver, heart, and kidney—rich sources of B12, B6, riboflavin, and folate—were highly valued and often eaten regularly in many cultures.[29] Fermented foods, sprouted grains, legumes, and seeds provided B1 (thiamine), B2 (riboflavin), B3 (niacin), and folate, while the inclusion of eggs, dairy, fish, and shellfish further supported B vitamin intake. Traditional preparation methods such as fermentation, nixtamalization (in corn-based cultures), and sourdough leavening improved bioavailability of these nutrients. Rather than isolating nutrients, traditional diets emphasized whole food synergy—how combinations of foods and preparation practices worked together to support vitality and well-being.[30]

Vitamin B12

If you're at the stage of life where perimenopause is on your radar or you're sending kids off to college, it's a good time to check your B12 levels. As we age, stomach acid and intrinsic factor naturally decrease, making it harder for the body to pull B12 from food. If you follow a vegan or vegetarian diet, you're also at a higher risk of deficiency since B12 is primarily found in animal products—so it's especially important to check your levels regularly.

Low B12 levels can show up in both mental and physical symptoms.[31] Mentally, a deficiency can contribute to depression, trouble with focus and memory, and increased irritability. Physically, signs may include pale skin, cracks or redness at the corners of the mouth (angular cheilitis), a swollen or smooth tongue, persistent fatigue, and loss of appetite. Digestive issues such as gas and diarrhea can also occur, along with neurological symptoms such as tingling or a "pins and needles" sensation in the feet.[32]

If you want to boost your intake, try adding these B12-rich foods to your diet:

- **Beef liver.** One of the richest sources of B12, though I won't pretend I love the taste. If liver isn't your thing, beef liver capsules can be an easier alternative. I once sprinkled beef liver powder on my smoothie alongside fish collagen—surf and turf at 8 AM!
- **Fortified nutritional yeast.** A cheesy-flavored topping that's great on popcorn or salads and, if fortified, is high in B12.
- **Oysters.** Fresh oysters are excellent, but if that's too adventurous, my dad swears by smoked oysters as an easy way to get more B12. Actually, he doesn't care about the B12 at all; he just really likes smoked oysters.

- **Fermented foods.** In communities with a traditional plant-based diet, B12 comes from tempeh, natto, and fermented grains.

Folate (Also Known as Vitamin B9)

Low folate levels can contribute to both mental and physical symptoms.[33] Mentally, a deficiency has been linked to depression, fatigue, irritability, and a decreased appetite as well as anemia. Physically, signs can include pale skin, a swollen or scarlet-red tongue, gingivitis, ridges on the nails, and a tingling or "pins and needles" sensation in the feet.[34]

Want to increase your folate intake? Here are some great options:

- **Mustard greens, collards, and turnip greens.** Sauté mustard greens, collards, or turnip greens with garlic and oil, simmer them in soups, or braise them slowly with broth and spices.
- **Lentils.** A folate powerhouse that's easy to mix into salads, omelets, or pasta dishes.
- **Chickpeas.** These are also high in folate, making hummus a great way to boost your intake.
- **Asparagus.** This vegetable is rich in folate, and it tastes great roasted with garlic and olive oil.
- **Plantains and sweet potatoes.** Roast plantains or sweet potatoes with spices, boil them for stews, or mash them with herbs and oil.

Vitamin B6

Vitamin B6 plays a key role in making neurotransmitters such as serotonin and dopamine, supporting your immune system, and helping your body process food into energy. When B6 levels are low, both your mood and your body can take a hit.[35] Mentally, deficiency may lead to depression, fatigue, irritability, and a lack of appetite, making it harder to stay motivated or feel like yourself. Physically, you might notice cracked or swollen corners of your mouth, pale skin, a red or sore tongue, or even dandruff. In more serious cases, B6 deficiency can lead to cavities, thick or scaly skin (a condition called pellagra), digestive issues such as gas or diarrhea, muscle twitching, or tingling in your feet.[36] Making sure you're getting enough B6—whether through food or supplements—can go a long way toward supporting your mood and overall well-being.

Looking to boost your vitamin B6 intake? Here are some easy ways to incorporate more B6-rich foods into your diet:

- **Lentils.** Simmer lentils into a spiced stew, toss them into salads or grain bowls, or cook them down with onions and herbs.
- **Turkey.** Great for sandwiches, salads, or a hearty protein option for dinner.
- **Wild salmon.** A nutrient-dense choice packed with both B6 and omega-3s.
- **Sesame seeds.** Toast sesame seeds and sprinkle them over rice, mix into sauces or dressings like tahini, or blend into spice mixes.
- **Russet potatoes with the skin.** Enjoy them as a baked potato or cut into wedges for homemade fries.
- **Cooked spinach.** Add it to omelets or soups or sauté it as a side dish.

Choosing the Right B Vitamin Supplement

If you're looking to support your B vitamin intake, a B complex supplement is usually a better choice than taking individual B vitamins. Most B complexes now include the active, more easily absorbed forms—such as methylcobalamin (B12), methylfolate (folate), and P5P (vitamin B6). These forms are especially helpful for people with certain genetic differences, such as MTHFR variants, which can make it harder to convert standard B vitamins into forms your body can actually use.

Methylation is an essential process that happens in every cell of your body. It supports everything from turning genes on and off to producing brain chemicals that support mood, stress response, and energy. It also plays a role in detoxification, inflammation, immune function, and cell repair.

This process depends on several nutrients including B vitamins, protein-based amino acids, and minerals such as zinc. If you're under chronic stress, dealing with inflammation, or have a genetic variation, your methylation process can slow down—and that can impact energy, mood, focus, and overall resilience.

To find out more about how your system methylates, you can work with a CNS or RD who is trained in nutrigenomics. They can review your genetic data, assess how your body processes B vitamins, and help you choose supplements that are better matched to your unique needs.

Turning Genes On and Off: The Power of Epigenetics

Epigenetics is the science of how our environment and lifestyle—things such as what we eat, how we move, how we manage stress, how well we sleep, and even the people we spend time with—can influence how our genes are turned on or off. This is powerful knowledge because it means our genes aren't fixed instructions—we have some say in how they're expressed.

One exciting area of epigenetics is the gut microbiome. The microbes in your gut aren't just passengers—they carry an estimated 5 million genes of their own, many of which can influence your health in positive ways. Supporting your gut health, as I'll describe in Chapters 8 and 9, creates a ripple effect, helping your genes work in your favor for better health in the long run.

Don't Ignore Iron

If you're feeling constantly fatigued, one of the first things I check is whether you're getting (and retaining) enough iron. I start by looking at your diet to see if you're consuming iron-rich foods, then I ask about your period—how often it comes, how long it lasts, and whether it's heavy. Finally, I take a look at your blood work. At a minimum, I check hemoglobin and MCV (mean corpuscular volume) to assess iron status, though my preference is to also check ferritin, the body's main iron storage protein. Unfortunately, ferritin isn't always included in routine lab tests.

Why is iron such a big deal? Because it helps carry oxygen through your body and fuels your energy production—two things your brain and body rely on every single day. When your iron levels dip, your brain may not get the oxygen it needs, which can leave you feeling foggy, unfocused, and emotionally off-balance.

Iron deficiency can lead to a range of mental and physical symptoms. Common mental health symptoms include brain fog, difficulty concentrating, low mood, and increased irritability. Physical symptoms may include fatigue, dizziness, pale skin, brittle nails, hair thinning, shortness of breath, and frequent cold hands and feet.[37]

Traditional diets were rich in iron from both plant and animal sources. Organ meats, red meat, and shellfish were often central to traditional meals and considered sacred or strengthening. Many traditional cultures also used cooking practices that supported iron absorption: pairing iron-rich foods with those high in vitamin C (such as wild greens, berries, or fermented vegetables) to enhance iron uptake from plant foods such as lentils, beans, and whole grains. Some communities cooked in cast-iron pots, which further increased the iron content of meals.

Want to boost your iron-rich food intake? Check out these options:

- **Amaranth grain.** Simmer amaranth grain into porridge, add it to soups for thickness, or use it as a hearty base for grain bowls.
- **Red meat.** This includes beef, lamb, pork. Dark meat poultry isn't red meat, but it has more iron than white meat.
- **Legumes.** Lentils, chickpeas, black beans, and soybeans are great vegetarian options.
- **Leafy greens.** Spinach, Swiss chard, and kale are excellent sources of plant-based iron.
- **Shellfish.** Clams, mussels, and oysters provide highly absorbable heme iron.
- **Tofu and tempeh.** These are great plant-based sources of iron and can be incorporated into a variety of meals.
- **Potatoes.** They contain iron, especially when eaten with the skin.

Pro tip: We absorb iron better when we eat it with sources of vitamin C. Consider using foods or condiments high in vitamin C with your iron-rich food. You might add red pepper strips, berries, or citrus. Or you could also experiment with adding condiments such as chimichurri, pico de gallo, amla chutney, lemon or lime pickle, and even some hot pepper sauces.

If you're looking for an easy way to boost iron in home-cooked meals, try using a cast-iron skillet when cooking acidic foods such as tomato sauce or chili—it helps leach small amounts of iron into your food. If you don't have a cast-iron skillet, or find it too heavy or cumbersome to use, another option is the Lucky Iron Fish (luckyironlife .com), a reusable iron cooking tool designed to add iron to soups, stews, and boiling water.

If lab work confirms an iron deficiency, food alone likely won't be enough to replenish your levels, and a supplement may be necessary. Because excessive iron can contribute to oxidative stress, supplementation should be done under the guidance of a healthcare provider. Research suggests that taking iron every other day (rather than daily) may improve absorption while reducing side effects such as constipation or nausea.

Zinc Deserves a Seat at the Table

If you've been feeling worn-out, scattered, or more emotionally reactive than usual, low zinc could be part of the picture. This essential mineral supports your mood, immune system, and the healing and repair of cells. Your body doesn't store much zinc, so it's important to get it regularly from the foods you eat.

Low zinc levels can show up in both your mood and your body. You might notice feeling more anxious or irritable, struggling to concentrate, or having a harder time coping with stress. Physically, signs can include feeling tired, getting sick more often, slower healing, thinning hair, brittle nails, or even changes in your sense of taste or smell.[38] Because zinc plays such an important role in immune health, skin repair, and brain function, keeping your levels steady really matters. If any of this sounds familiar, it may be worth adding more zinc-rich foods to your meals or checking in with a healthcare provider about supplementation.

Global diets naturally support zinc intake through animal-based foods such as red meat, shellfish (especially oysters), and organ meats—some of the most bioavailable sources of zinc. In plant-based traditions, zinc from legumes, seeds (such as pumpkin and sesame), nuts, and whole grains was emphasized.

Here are some zinc-rich foods to consider adding to your diet:

- **Oysters.** The best natural source of zinc, though not to everyone's liking.
- **Fermented bean pastes.** Add miso to soups or marinades, mix ogiri into stews or sauces for umami depth, and eat natto with rice, mustard, or soy sauce.
- **Red meat.** Beef, lamb, and pork are great, widely available options.
- **Poultry.** Chicken and turkey, especially dark meat, contain good amounts of zinc.
- **Pumpkin seeds and other seeds.** A fantastic plant-based zinc source; toss them into salads, yogurt, or smoothies.
- **Lentils and chickpeas.** Great for plant-based eaters looking to increase zinc intake.

If dietary intake isn't enough or lab results confirm a deficiency, supplementation may be needed. Long-term zinc supplements should always be taken with caution—too much can interfere with copper absorption and may cause nausea or digestive upset.

Food for Thought

Before moving on, take a moment to reflect on your current eating patterns. How do they align with the nutrients we've discussed? Are there gaps in your intake? Have you noticed any symptoms of nutrient insufficiency in yourself?

If so, remember—this isn't about shame or blame. It's simply information, an opportunity to learn and adjust. Nutrition is a lifelong practice, not a test you need to pass. What matters is that you're paying attention and open to making small, meaningful shifts that work with your nervous system, not against it.

The goal of the food part of the FIGS protocol isn't to overwhelm you with the idea that you need to optimize every single nutrient. Instead, it's about noticing where your body may need support and learning how to gently add in what's missing—without disrupting your sense of safety.

CHAPTER 6

I Is for Inflammation: Trauma Drives It; How Do You Want to Reduce It?

> The body and mind are sensitive and react to regimes of oppression.
>
> —Johanna Hedva, *Sick Woman Theory*

I probably don't need to convince you that trauma-driven inflammation contributes to physical diseases—everything from cardiovascular disease and diabetes to fibromyalgia and autoimmune conditions. Even higher rates of asthma have been linked to early-life trauma.

But when you've heard about inflammation, chances are it was framed as something caused by poor diet or lack of exercise—hence the emphasis on anti-inflammatory diets and lifestyle changes. While diet and movement can influence inflammation, I want you to look at your trauma history as a factor that has predisposed you to inflammatory disease. Before we dive into ways to combat inflammation in the next chapter, we need to take a step back and examine how it shows up in your life.

Dr. Robin Ross, a psychologist mentor of mine, once asked me, "How does inflammation feel in the body?" The only answer I could give was "It feels like crap." Acute inflammation—the swelling and soreness you feel after stepping on a nail—is pretty straightforward. However, chronic systemic inflammation, the kind that often follows trauma, is much more insidious. It doesn't just cause pain and swelling; it can manifest as fatigue, exhaustion, difficulty sleeping, muscle soreness, depression, anxiety, and even digestive issues.

When most people try to improve their health, they assume that simply eating better or exercising more is all they need to feel good. And while those things can help, they don't tell the whole story. If trauma has rewired your nervous system to constantly scan for danger, your body is likely in a chronic state of inflammation—whether you're eating blueberries or not.

This is why disease is not your fault. If you're living in an abusive household, no amount of kale or turmeric is going to fully offset the impact of ongoing stress on your immune system. If your nervous system is stuck in survival mode, inflammatory cytokines flood your system, keeping your body in a constant state of alarm.

Trauma Increases Inflammation, Predisposing Us to Disease

If you've experienced trauma, there is a huge likelihood that you've felt the effects of inflammation in your body. Traumatic events activate the body's stress response systems—especially the sympathetic nervous system (which prepares the body to fight or flee) and the HPA axis (a hormone-regulating system that helps the body cope with stress). These systems influence how the immune system behaves.

The Mind-Body Link: How Stress Talks to Your Immune System

The field of psychoneuroimmunology (PNI) explores the powerful connection between the mind and body. It shows how chronic stress—whether emotional or physiological—can disrupt key biological systems, including the nervous system, immune function, hormone balance, and even the gut microbiome. These systems are in constant, two-way communication, and when one is out of balance, it can affect the others. PNI shows us how deeply our thoughts, feelings, and stress levels can shape both our mental and physical health.

In a healthy, short-term stress response, the body releases glucocorticoids—stress hormones such as cortisol—that help keep inflammation in check. But when stress is ongoing or unresolved, the body can get stuck in a defensive state. In this state, the sympathetic nervous system stays revved up, and instead of calming inflammation, the body starts producing more of it.

Pro-inflammatory chemicals called cytokines (such as IL-6, TNF-α, and IL-17) increase while anti-inflammatory messengers (such as IL-4 and IL-10) decrease.[1] These danger signals can even travel to the brain—either through the vagus nerve or by crossing a weakened blood-brain barrier—where they activate immune cells in the brain called microglia. This creates neuroinflammation, which has been linked to many mental health challenges, including anxiety, depression, and brain fog.

Some people are able to return to a state of ventral regulation after a stressful event. But for many—especially those with trauma—these stress responses and the resulting inflammation can become long-term patterns, affecting both mental and physical health over time.

Let's take a closer look at the data. If you have an inflammatory condition (which, to be honest, includes most diseases), you may have been made to feel like it's your fault—that if only you had eaten better, exercised more, or tried harder, you wouldn't be sick. That's simply not true.

In the functional medicine model of nutrition that I was taught, we often explore the antecedents, triggers, and mediators of disease. Antecedents are predisposing factors—things that set the stage for disease, such as a parent smoking in your home growing up. Triggers are the events that "turn on" a disease, such as a bout of food poisoning leading to IBS. Mediators are the ongoing factors that keep a disease going, such as chronic work stress contributing to high cortisol and systemic inflammation.

Stress from trauma can act as *all three*. Here's how:

- **As an antecedent.** Trauma creates long-term changes in how your nervous system and immune system function. For example, a child who grows up in a high-conflict household may develop a chronically activated stress response, making their body more vulnerable to inflammatory conditions such as autoimmune disease, heart disease, or IBS later in life.
- **As a trigger.** A trigger doesn't have to be just a single traumatic event—it can be a chronic illness, a period of intense stress, or even an infection that tips the body over a threshold. For example, someone who experiences a violent

assault, a major surgery, or a long stretch of burnout may develop inflammatory conditions such as fibromyalgia or autoimmune diseases, even if they had no previous signs of illness.

- **As a mediator.** Even after the original trauma has passed, the body can stay stuck in survival mode. Ongoing hypervigilance, sleep disturbances, emotional numbing, and chronic anxiety all act as constant stressors on the body's systems. Instead of being able to fully rest and repair, the body remains on high alert, like a guard who never goes off duty. This constant low-level stress fuels inflammation over time, wearing down the immune system, disrupting gut health, throwing off hormone balance, and keeping chronic conditions—such as autoimmune flares, gut dysfunction, or mood disorders— alive and active.

What's important to understand is that the stress response doesn't require something to happen *right now*—it can be activated just as powerfully by a stressful thought or memory as by a real-time event. The amygdala, our brain's threat detection center, doesn't distinguish between an actual danger and a recalled or imagined one. When it senses a threat, it signals the hypothalamus to launch the body's stress response, triggering a cascade that includes the release of stress hormones and inflammatory chemicals. When this happens chronically, it suppresses the calming influence of the vagus nerve, making it harder to combat inflammation.

Here are some of the diseases linked to chronic inflammation, many of which have also been connected to trauma:

- Alzheimer's disease
- Asthma

- Cancer
- Cardiovascular disease (including atherosclerosis, heart attack, stroke)
- Chronic fatigue syndrome
- Chronic obstructive pulmonary disease (COPD)
- Depression and anxiety disorders
- Diabetes
- Endometriosis
- Fibromyalgia
- Gout
- Hypertension
- Inflammatory bowel diseases (including Crohn's disease and ulcerative colitis)
- Metabolic dysfunction-associated steatotic liver disease (MASLD)
- Metabolic syndrome
- Multiple sclerosis
- Psoriasis
- Rheumatoid arthritis
- Sleep apnea

As we move through the rest of this chapter, we're going to look at a few specific ways trauma can drive inflammation. These are just examples—they don't cover every kind of trauma, and they're not the only reasons you might be dealing with inflammation. Take a peek at the image below for even more possibilities. Your body's story is unique, and chances are, more than one factor has played a role.

In the next chapter, we'll talk about how to start calming inflammation—not with guilt trips or unrealistic expectations, but with small, doable shifts that help your body feel safer over time. For now, just know this: if you're living with an inflammatory condition, it didn't happen because you "failed" at healthy eating or exercise. Your history matters. What you've lived through matters. And there's a lot more right with you than wrong.

MANY Factors Cause Inflammation
Trauma that happened in the past
Trauma that is happening currently
Financial instability
Marginalization and racism
Safety in relationships at home and work
Loneliness
Chronic, toxic levels of stress
Chronic diseases
Infections such as COVID, Lyme, or Epstein-Barr
Smoking, alcohol and drug use
Dental problems
Sleep problems
Lack of physical activity
Excessive physical activity
Environmental toxins
Lack of connection with nature

Focus on What Feels Modifiable
Social connection
Get into nature
Breathe
Explore mindfulness
Get good sleep
Move your body
Eat anti-inflammatory foods

Many things drive inflammation—some we can't control, and some we can. Rather than blaming yourself for what's outside your power, focus on small, supportive shifts that feel possible right now. Healing starts with what is modifiable.

Did You Experience Trauma as a Child?

Fibromyalgia (FM) is a chronic pain condition that affects millions of people—and for a long time, researchers have suspected that early life trauma might play a role in why it develops. But until recently, we didn't have a clear picture of exactly what kinds of childhood experiences might be linked to FM.

One study helped shed some light on it. Researchers compared the childhood experiences of people with fibromyalgia to over 400,000 people surveyed by the Centers for Disease Control (CDC). The results? People with FM were much more likely to have experienced tough things growing up compared to the general population.[2]

- Nearly half (47 percent) of FM patients grew up with a depressed or mentally ill caregiver, compared to just 15 percent of the general population.

- 53 percent were verbally abused by their parents, more than double the rate found in the CDC's survey.

- 42 percent of FM patients reported being hit by their parents compared to only 10 percent of the general population.

- One in four FM patients (26 percent) were sexually abused as children compared to only 9 percent of the general population.

- 34 percent experienced attempted sexual abuse, and 21 percent were forced into sex by an adult, far exceeding national averages.

This study doesn't mean that everyone with fibromyalgia has these exact experiences—or that these are the only traumas that can lead to inflammation and chronic illness. Far from it. But it does give us a powerful window into how childhood adversity can leave deep imprints on the body, especially on how the nervous system and pain pathways develop.

And FM isn't the only condition linked to early trauma. We'll keep unpacking this idea as we move through the next sections because understanding where inflammation comes from helps us figure out how to support healing, too.

Have You Experienced Sexual Harassment or Sexual Assault?

A recent study looked at 304 nonsmoking midlife women and found something important: women who had experienced sexual harassment at work had significantly higher odds of having high blood pressure and poor sleep compared to those who hadn't been harassed. And women who had a history of sexual assault? They were far more likely to struggle with depression, anxiety, and really disrupted sleep.[3]

Even after researchers accounted for other health factors—such as income, overall health, and lifestyle differences—the link between trauma and these health issues stayed strong. This tells us that it's not just about circumstances or bad luck. Trauma itself leaves a real imprint on the body.

Why does this matter? Because high blood pressure, poor sleep, anxiety, and depression all have something in common: They're connected to systemic inflammation. Trauma keeps the nervous system on high alert, stuck in a hypervigilant, fight-or-flight mode. The women in this study who had experienced assault had significantly higher rates of anxiety and poor sleep—two big red flags that the stress response never got the message it was safe to turn off.

The findings around workplace harassment were just as eye-opening. Even though harassment is often brushed off as "just part of the job" (ugh, don't even get me started), the reality is that women who had been harassed at work had higher blood pressure—a clear sign of chronic stress. And high blood pressure isn't just uncomfortable; it's one of the biggest risk factors for heart disease—which, by the way, is still the leading cause of death for women.

Trauma isn't just something we "get over." It reshapes the body's systems—often in ways we can't see right away but that absolutely matter over time.

Do You Experience Racism?

A large meta-analysis pulled together data from lots of studies and found something we absolutely can't ignore: Experiencing racism has a real, measurable impact on health. People who reported facing racism were more likely to struggle with mental health issues, have higher blood pressure, and show signs of something called allostatic load, which basically means their bodies were worn down from being stuck in a constant state of stress.[4]

This kind of chronic stress builds up when someone is exposed to ongoing threats, such as discrimination, microaggressions, or systemic inequality. It keeps the body stuck in survival mode, flooding it with stress hormones such as cortisol and adrenaline. These hormones are useful when you need to escape a short-term danger—but when they're activated all the time? They start causing damage, especially to the cardiovascular system.

One of the most striking things this study found was that people who experienced racism had higher blood pressure, even after researchers accounted for other factors such as income, diet, and exercise. And it wasn't just regular blood pressure readings; it showed up in ambulatory blood pressure, which tracks your blood pressure throughout the day. That means even when people seemed calm on the outside, their bodies were still carrying the chronic stress underneath.

And it's not just blood pressure. The study also showed that racism takes a toll on mental health:

- People who experienced discrimination had higher rates of anxiety and depression.
- Poor sleep—a classic sign of chronic stress—was much more common among those exposed to racism.
- Even people who didn't already have high blood pressure were more likely to develop it over time if they reported high levels of discrimination.

Bottom line? Racism isn't just something that hurts emotionally; it leaves an ongoing, lasting imprint on the body. And it's something we need to name, acknowledge, and address when we're talking about trauma, stress, and healing.

Have You Been in a Challenging Relationship?

When we think about challenging relationships, especially abusive or controlling ones, we usually focus on emotional damage—and for good reason. But what often gets overlooked is that these relationships aren't just bad for your mental health. They can have serious, lasting effects on your physical health too, especially your heart.

Researchers have found that the stress of ongoing relationship conflict—such as emotional manipulation, constant criticism, or feeling isolated—can leave a real biological imprint. Stress hormones stay elevated. Inflammatory pathways get activated. Over time, your body absorbs that tension, leading to changes you can't just "think" your way out of.

In one recent study, women who had experienced intimate partner violence (IPV) were far more likely to report chest pain, heart palpitations, anxiety, and PTSD. But it wasn't just how they felt emotionally; their bodies also showed clear signs of increased inflammation, a major risk factor for heart disease.[5]

And it's not just IPV. Decades of research show that the quality of your close relationships shapes your immune system too:[6]

- Supportive, trusting relationships are linked to lower inflammation and better long-term health.
- Conflict-heavy or isolating relationships are linked to higher inflammation—even when controlling for factors such as smoking, diet, and exercise.
- Relational stress—whether from arguments, control, or emotional withdrawal—can directly trigger inflammatory responses in the body through stress hormones such as norepinephrine.
- Depression, often worsened by toxic relationships, can amplify inflammation even further by disrupting sleep, appetite, and physical resilience.

Scientists have found that relationship stress takes a real toll on the body in two big ways. First, it can directly fire up the nervous system's stress response and kick the immune system into an inflammatory state. Second, it can work more indirectly—by fueling depression, messing with sleep, stirring up emotional stress, and making it harder to take care of yourself. Over time, both paths can leave your body stuck in a constant state of inflammation, draining your energy and increasing your risk for all kinds of health issues.

It's not just your imagination. Challenging and toxic relationships change your body.

And when it comes to your health, the aftermath can be just as real—and just as important to heal—as the emotional wounds.

If you've been through an unsupportive relationship, it's not "all in your head." Your nervous system, your heart, and your entire body have been carrying that load. Healing means tending to all of it.

Do You Work the Night Shift?

At first glance, working the night shift may not seem like a traumatic experience. After all, many people voluntarily choose or adapt to working overnight. But when I've asked night shift workers if they find their work traumatic, most say yes—immediately. Even those who don't consciously label it as trauma often describe feeling exhausted, isolated, or emotionally worn down. Their bodies feel the strain, even if their minds try to push through it.

We're learning more and more that when your body's natural sleep-wake cycle gets thrown off—what's called circadian disruption —it doesn't just mess with your energy levels. It can seriously impact your health too. Disrupted circadian rhythms are now linked to higher risks of high blood pressure, heart disease, and chronic inflammation.

One recent study looked at more than 350,000 adults in the UK Biobank and found some pretty clear connections between sleep patterns, shift work, and blood pressure:[7]

- People who worked night shifts were a lot more likely to have high blood pressure.
- Those stuck on permanent night shifts had an even stronger risk compared to people who rotated shifts or had mixed schedules.
- It wasn't just working nights; both sleeping too little (fewer than five hours) and sleeping too much (more than nine hours) made things worse for night-shift workers' blood pressure.

In short, when your sleep gets out of sync with your natural rhythms, your heart and immune system can pay the price.

Even if you *feel* like you've adjusted to a night schedule, your body hasn't. We are biologically wired to sync with natural light and dark cycles. When you work through the night and sleep during the day, your internal clock gets thrown out of alignment, keeping your body in a state of chronic stress without you even realizing it. This disruption doesn't just affect your energy. It ripples out into multiple areas of health, including your mood.[8]

And it's not just your brain on a schedule; your gut is too. Recent research shows that your gut microbiome—the community of microbes living inside you—follows its own circadian rhythm. When that rhythm is thrown off, it can lead to gut imbalance (dysbiosis), increased gut permeability ("leaky gut"), and higher levels of systemic inflammation.[9]

The bigger picture? Trauma doesn't always look like a major event. Sometimes it's the slow erosion of safety over time—like living out of sync with your body's natural needs.

Simple Swaps to Support Your Body's Healing Environment

Your mood isn't just shaped by your thoughts or what happened today; it's also influenced by your hormones, your immune system, and even what your body is exposed to in the environment. Some everyday chemicals, called *endocrine disruptors,* can throw off your body's natural balance. These are found in things such as plastics, personal care products, and even furniture or household dust. Over time, they may interfere with mood-regulating hormones, increase brain inflammation, and make it harder for your nervous system to feel safe and calm—especially if you're healing from trauma.

You can't control every exposure. Pollution, food packaging, or the water coming from your tap may be out of your hands. But some small, doable changes—like using a glass water bottle, switching to fragrance-free products, or avoiding microwaving plastic—can reduce your body's load. It's not about being perfect. It's about lowering stressors where you can so your body and brain have more space to rest and recover.[10]

Do You Feel Lonely?

Loneliness doesn't just hurt emotionally; it takes a real toll on the body too. Research keeps uncovering just how closely loneliness and inflammation are linked. Just like your body responds to a cut or injury with inflammation, it turns out emotional injuries can spark a similar biological response.

In one study of middle-aged adults, loneliness was strongly associated with higher levels of inflammatory markers such as IL-6, fibrinogen, and C-reactive protein (CRP).[11] And the effect seems even stronger for people who are particularly sensitive to social disconnection; they show bigger spikes in inflammation when they face psychological stress.[12]

And you don't have to actually be alone to feel lonely. On the surface, you're surrounded by conversation, laughter, and activity. But inside, you feel disconnected, unseen, or even invisible. It's not the physical presence of others that relieves loneliness; it's the feeling of being known, understood, and emotionally connected.

Here are ways you can feel lonely in a crowd:

- You don't feel emotionally safe enough to share your real thoughts or feelings.
- You're masking or performing a version of yourself that doesn't match how you really feel inside.

- The people around you don't seem to notice or care about what you're going through.
- You sense that you don't truly belong or that if you did show your authentic self, you might be rejected.
- There's an emotional mismatch between you and the group: Everyone else seems carefree or connected while you feel distant or weighed down.

Loneliness isn't about how many people are around you; it's about how connected you feel to them. You can have ten people at your side and still feel completely alone if there's no emotional bridge between you.

And because your nervous system is wired for connection, when that bridge feels broken or absent, your body registers it as a kind of danger—even if everything looks "fine" on the outside. That's why social disconnection can trigger real physiological stress responses, including inflammation.

Here's something even more surprising: Inflammation doesn't just *respond* to how you feel—it can actually *shape* how you behave. When you go through adversity, your body kicks off a biological process known as the conserved transcriptional response to adversity (CTRA). Think of it as an ancient survival mode. When your brain perceives danger (such as isolation or rejection), it ramps up genes that promote inflammation, getting your body ready to heal if you get hurt. But it also dials down the genes that fight off viruses, making you more vulnerable to infections over time.

CTRA is mostly triggered by social disconnection. In simple terms, when you feel isolated, your body treats it like a serious threat, releasing stress hormones and inflammatory messengers into your system. Thanks to research from the field of human social genomics, we now know that experiences such as loneliness, rejection, and trauma don't just *feel* painful; they actually turn on genes that prepare the body for physical survival.

> Research on adult attachment shows that the quality of our close relationships—and how safe we feel within them—has a powerful impact on both mental and physical health. Individuals with insecure attachment styles—particularly those with high attachment anxiety or avoidance—were more likely to experience emotional struggles such as loneliness, depression, and anxiety. These emotional states don't just affect how we feel; they also activate biological stress responses, including inflammation. Insecure attachment can train the nervous system to see social situations as threatening, which may contribute to a persistent state of inflammation, such as the one triggered by the CTRA response.[12,13]

When you catch a cold or the flu, your body kicks off a short burst of inflammation to help you fight it off. Once the illness passes, the inflammation usually settles back down. But if your body is already primed for chronic inflammation—often because of trauma—that response doesn't just turn off. It lingers, and over time, it starts influencing your emotions and behavior in powerful ways.

When inflammation becomes a long-term pattern, it's not just your physical health that's affected; it can change how you feel, how you connect with others, and even how you move through the world. This is called sickness behavior, and it often shows up as fatigue and low energy, loss of interest in activities you used to enjoy, changes in appetite, and pulling away from social interactions.

These shifts aren't "all in your head." They're driven by inflammatory cytokines—chemical messengers that send danger signals to

your brain. Inflammation can also disrupt the production of serotonin, a key chemical that helps regulate mood and motivation. The
result? You might find yourself withdrawing from people, feeling
disconnected from things you once loved, and struggling to find the
energy to take care of yourself.

Chronic inflammation can shift behavior in ways that push you away from the very support systems that can help you heal.

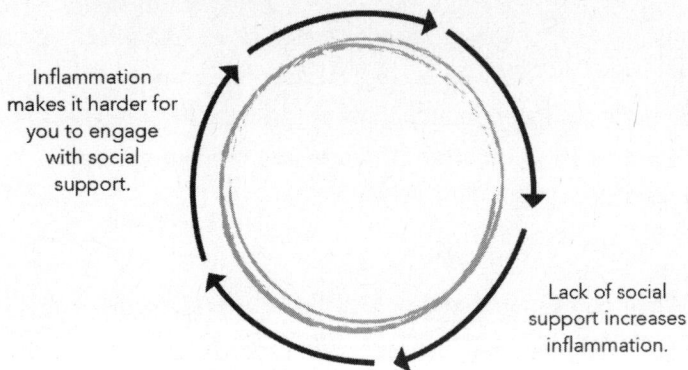

Inflammation makes it harder for you to engage with social support.

Lack of social support increases inflammation.

When inflammation is high, it becomes harder to seek out or receive connection. But disconnection itself worsens inflammation, deepening the spiral.

At first, this withdrawal actually serves a purpose—it's your
body's way of conserving energy to focus on healing. But if you stay
in this state for too long, what started as a protective response can
spiral into something more damaging, such as chronic depression,
deep isolation, and even more inflammation.

In other words, trauma doesn't just leave emotional scars; it can
rewire your biology in ways that shape how you live and connect,
even long after the original event has passed.

So What's Next?

If you're starting to realize just how many ways inflammation can take hold in the body, you're not alone. It's a lot. And it's complex.

Some sources of inflammation are simply out of our control. These are the nonmodifiable triggers, meaning you didn't cause them and you can't magically erase them, such as past trauma, early-life adversity, and systemic stressors such as racism, poverty, or discrimination.

These experiences leave a real imprint on the body. If you've lived through them, it makes sense that your nervous system and immune system may be on high alert. It's not a personal failure; it's a biological response to surviving in a world that wasn't always safe.

But—and this is a really important "but"—there are also things you *can* influence. They're not about pretending the hard things never happened. They're about building small pockets of support for your body and nervous system right now, in the life you're living today.

In the next chapter, we'll talk about these modifiable factors— things you can gently shift to help your body find its way back toward steadiness:

- Creating more moments of ventral regulation—even tiny ones—through practices that help you feel grounded and safe
- Strengthening connections with friends, family, pets, or community
- Supporting better sleep and daily rhythms to give your body a predictable, soothing routine
- Spending time in nature to calm your stress response and lower inflammation naturally

- Using nutrition, movement, and medical support in ways that meet you where you are, not where you "should" be

You may not be able to erase the inflammation caused by childhood trauma. You may not be able to stop the ongoing inflammation triggered by systemic stress. You may not be able to change the inflammation sparked by an abusive workplace.

But you *can* modify the ways you support your nervous system today.

CHAPTER 7

You Can Calm the Fire: How to Lower Inflammation and Support Healing

Every symptom has a story to tell.
We just have to listen.

—Dr. Gabor Maté

You might be surprised to learn that 60 to 80 percent of all primary care physician visits are due to the wear and tear on the body due to stress and trauma.[1] Now, I'm not proposing that when we have a hard day, we march right off to the doctor's office. Let's all collectively imagine the look on the doctors' faces! But too many hard days in succession can lead to the immune system becoming dysregulated, resulting in increased cold and flu infections, as well as worsening other chronic diseases.[2]

The more time you spend in a regulated state, the more opportunities your body has to rest, repair, and heal. If you're looking for more ways to build ventral regulation into your daily life, I highly recommend Deb Dana's book *Anchored: How to Befriend Your Nervous System Using Polyvagal Theory*—it's full of practical, compassionate tools.[3]

In the last chapter, we explored how trauma-driven inflammation can take hold in the body, contributing to both physical and mental health challenges. Now, we turn our attention to what we can do about it. While some factors influencing inflammation are outside our control—such as past trauma, systemic stressors, and early-life adversity—there are many modifiable factors that we can shift in the present to help calm inflammation and support healing.

This chapter isn't about perfection. It's about creating shifts—small, meaningful ones—that help your body feel safer over time. Some strategies, such as spending time in nature or strengthening social connections, help bring calming, regulated energy back into your system. Others, such as going to the dentist or addressing hidden sources of stress, may not feel soothing in the moment but create longer-term safety and resilience.

Get a Primary Care Provider

If you don't already have a primary care provider (PCP), this is your gentle nudge to get one. I know that finding a doctor, making the appointment, and navigating the healthcare system isn't anyone's idea of a good time. But it matters. And here's why.

So many of the health challenges you may be facing such as inflammation, fatigue, or gut issues intersect with things that need medical support. For example, thyroid disorders, autoimmune conditions, sleep apnea, and even anemia can mimic or worsen trauma-related symptoms. A good primary care provider can help rule out, diagnose, and manage those issues. Here's what I recommend when looking for a primary care provider:

- Start by asking around. Friends, family, or trusted providers such as your therapist might have referrals.
- Check online reviews but read between the lines. Sometimes complaints are about things such as wait times rather than the quality of care.
- When you call to schedule, ask if the provider is comfortable working with patients who have trauma histories or complex chronic health conditions. How the front desk responds can tell you a lot.
- You're allowed to switch. If the first provider you meet isn't a good fit, it's okay to try someone else. You're not "difficult" for advocating for yourself.

I get it, "find a primary care provider" isn't the sexiest wellness advice out there. It's way less exciting than some of the other options in this chapter. But honestly? It might be the most important thing on the list. You need a solid teammate in your corner—someone who can help you navigate labs, diagnoses, and referrals. All the anti-inflammatory foods in the world won't replace having medical support when you need it. This work is hard enough without trying to fly solo. Find someone who can walk alongside you.

Focus on Social Connection

Healthy relationships are at the heart of our emotional and physical well-being. They give us a sense of safety and connection that helps regulate our nervous system. When we grow up with consistent, supportive caregivers, we naturally develop secure attachment patterns—internal templates that help us trust others, seek support, and feel soothed in connection.

But when those early relationships are marked by neglect, rejection, or chaos—especially in the context of trauma—our nervous system adapts to prioritize survival. Some people develop anxious attachment, feeling constantly on edge about being abandoned or not being good enough. Others move toward avoidant attachment, learning to protect themselves by downplaying their need for closeness and relying only on themselves.

Attachment theory was originally developed by British psychoanalyst John Bowlby, who described how we form the internal blueprints for relationships based on our experiences with caregivers early in life. These unconscious blueprints show up in later relationships too, especially in times of stress. These patterns aren't personal failings—they're survival strategies that made sense at the time.

Research shows that insecure attachment—especially attachment anxiety—is closely linked to more intense PTSD symptoms, particularly when trauma happens early in life. People with high attachment anxiety often have stronger physical reactions when recalling traumatic memories and tend to replay those memories frequently, sometimes intentionally and sometimes not. This constant reactivation can make traumatic memories feel even more vivid and overwhelming, fueling the severity of PTSD symptoms.[4]

Avoidant attachment shows up differently. People with avoidant patterns may not rehash traumatic memories as often, but they tend to suppress emotions and keep others at a distance. While this can create a sense of control in the short term, it also limits emotional support and can leave them feeling disconnected, isolated, or emotionally numb over time.

When Inflammation Makes Connection Harder

Remember, inflammation can also affect our ability to be social. Studies show that people experiencing inflammation often withdraw socially, feel more anxious or irritable, and have a harder time trusting others.

Understanding how attachment patterns shape our response to trauma helps reframe symptoms—not as weaknesses but as adaptations to a world that didn't feel safe. The good news is that attachment isn't fixed. With time, support, and new experiences of safety and connection, our nervous system can begin to trust again—and healing can happen in relationship.

Many of my clients who have experienced trauma describe a deep desire for connection while also feeling unable to seek it out. As Deb Dana writes in *Polyvagal Theory in Therapy,* "Clients will often say that they needed connection but there was no one in their life who was safe, so after a while they stopped looking."[5] Even when someone stops consciously searching for support, their nervous system doesn't stop craving it.

From a polyvagal perspective, the need for coregulation is wired into us, but when past relationships have been a source of harm or stress, reaching out for connection can feel risky. Recognizing this tension—between wanting connection and fearing it—can be the first step in learning how to rebuild trust and safety in relationships.

A growing body of research shows that strong, positive relationships help protect us against inflammation. One study of US adults found that while support from others can be protective, stress from family, friends, or social interactions can actually increase inflammation—and not just a little. In fact, feeling strained in relationships was a stronger predictor of stress and inflammation than the benefits of social support.[6]

In other words: When relationships feel heavy, it's not always easy—or even possible—to reach out for help. And if you've experienced trauma early in life, especially in your relationships with caregivers, your nervous system might be wired to withdraw as a form of protection.

So where can you start if relationships feel hard or overwhelming? One surprisingly powerful option is to focus on building a sense of purpose.

In one study, researchers found that having a strong sense of meaning—what's called *eudaimonic well-being*—could actually buffer some of the inflammatory effects of loneliness.[7] Purpose doesn't have to be something grand or dramatic. It can be built, one small step at a time.

If you want to explore this, try asking yourself:

- What makes me feel useful?
- Who or what do I want to show up for?

You might find purpose by journaling about what you want to contribute to the world, volunteering in your community, planting a garden, or simply helping a neighbor. Start with what you care about and follow where it leads.

If you're looking to rebuild or strengthen human connection, here are a few gentle ideas clients have found helpful:

- **Start small.** Begin with low-stakes interactions like greeting a neighbor or chatting briefly with a cashier. Hold a door for someone or send a "thinking of you" text to a friend. Smile at a dog or wave to your neighbor.

- **Set realistic goals.** Instead of aiming to attend large social gatherings, reach out to one person a week or attend a small event.
- **Plan short interactions.** If longer social engagements feel daunting, plan a fifteen-minute chat or walk around the block with a friend.
- **Put an event on your calendar.** Check out your local public library for movie screenings and book clubs. You can delete it later if need be. Remember, this is all about small steps.

And if people still feel too hard? That's okay too. Animals, especially dogs, can offer a powerful bridge back to connection. Research shows that dogs help regulate stress, ease anxiety, and create attachment bonds similar to the ones we form with caregivers. If you're feeling disconnected from the human world, a dog's steady companionship—the nudges, tail wags, and quiet presence—can be a way to start feeling safe again. Sometimes regulation begins not with a deep conversation, but with a wagging tail and a soft nudge that says, "You're not alone."[8]

Get into Nature

Rejoice nature lovers. This one's for you. Researchers have found that the more pleasant experiences you have in nature, the greater the anti-inflammatory response in the body. There have been many studies linking time in nature to anti-inflammatory effects, and most don't require a three-mile hike to reap the benefits. From spending time near water, to forest bathing, to gardening, to engaging with nature helps lessen inflammatory cytokines and stress hormones.

And if you're not an outdoors person, don't worry. You can also garden indoors and receive many of the same anti-inflammatory benefits of going outside. One study conducted by the University of Helsinki[9] showed that just one month of indoor gardening using a microbially rich soil was associated with higher levels of anti-inflammatory molecules in the blood.

So, while you could take the approach of Cheryl Strayed, author of *Wild*, and hike the 2,650-mile Pacific Coast Trail (!), you don't need to choose an option quite so radical. Consider if any of these ideas below resonate with you. You also don't need to commit forever; you can just choose something to do today:

- **Take a short walk around the block.** Just ten to fifteen minutes in nature can reduce stress and inflammation. Research shows *shinrin-yoku*, or forest bathing, reduces stress hormones, including cortisol, adrenaline, and noradrenaline while also increasing activation of the parasympathetic nervous system—all of which support balance of the autonomic nervous system.[10]

- **Sit by water.** This is one of my personal favorites. We have a large local pond that has a nearby parking lot overlooking the water. Folks, I often don't even get out of the car. Just sitting there watching the water helps me feel better. Studies have shown that looking at bodies of water can help reduce heart rate and blood pressure while increasing relaxation.[11]

- **Grow a garden.** If you have outdoor space, spend a little time tending to plants or flowers. If not, consider starting an indoor garden with herbs or small plants. I recently bought a tiny basil plant from the grocery store and planted it in one of my extra mugs! You could even start plants from cut herbs or vegetables you use to cook. Gardening is a great way to connect with nature, with a meta-analysis revealing it offers various benefits to our health, including reductions in anxiety and depression symptoms, while increasing quality of life and sense of community.[12, 13]

- **Take a sunshine break.** Perhaps you live in a place blessed by abundant year-round sunshine. Not so here in the Midwest in winter, but there is a day in the early spring that I always try to capture. It's the first day you can be outside comfortably without a winter coat when the sun is shining and there is usually a light breeze. This is my absolute favorite weather feeling: When the sun warms my skin, it just seems like the entire world is opening up again. This is because exposure to sunlight has a positive correlation with mental health.[14, 15]

- **Listen to nature sounds.** Open the windows and listen to the birds singing and the leaves blowing in the breeze. You can also listen to a nature sounds app. In one study, participants reported feeling more comfortable and relaxed and experienced fewer negative feelings.[16]

Explore Breathing Exercises and Mindfulness

Using your breath is a free, readily accessible tool to lessen inflammation. However, for people with a history of trauma, breathing exercises can feel anything but calming. For example, someone who experienced panic attacks in the past may associate the sensation of deep breathing with the onset of those episodes—#noticebreathing #gaspingforair. Another person who endured medical trauma, choking, or being physically held down might experience an increased sense of danger when focusing on their breath because the very act of tuning into their body brings them back to moments when breath was not safe or in their control.

Stillness itself can feel unsafe for many people who have experienced trauma, especially if hypervigilance and staying on the edge was once protective. Instead of calm, paying attention to the breath brings a shift to a survival state. If this resonates with you, and you want to explore breathwork and mindfulness practices, I'd highly recommend David A. Treleaven's *Trauma-Sensitive Mindfulness* as a guide to safe exploration.[17]

Breathwork Isn't New: Honoring Ancestral Practices

Many somatic practices now used for nervous system regulation, such as breathwork, or rhythmic movement, have been used throughout global cultures for generations. These practices have been heavily commercialized. If it feels supportive and you have access, there are apps that will guide you in breathwork practices. If you have breathwork traditions in your ancestry that feel good to you, do those instead.

If breathwork feels supportive to you, there are good reasons to pursue it as a way to help you lessen inflammation. In one study, researchers wanted to see if specific breathing techniques could lower the levels of certain substances in saliva that indicate inflammation. They divided twenty healthy volunteers into two groups: one group practiced the breathing exercises with a trained instructor while the other group read a book for the same amount of time. They collected saliva samples before and after the exercises to measure different markers that show inflammation.

The results showed that the group practicing yogic breathing had lower levels of three specific markers linked to inflammation in their saliva compared to the reading group.[18] This means that doing certain breathing exercises may help reduce stress and inflammation in the body. If you have a history of panic attacks or psychosis, I'd recommend exploring breathwork with a trusted professional. Here are a few of my favorite breathing practices:

- **4-7-8 breath.** This simple breathing technique can be a powerful tool to help your body shift into a more relaxed state. To try it, inhale gently through your nose for a count of four, hold your breath for a count of seven, and then exhale slowly through your mouth for a count of eight. In one study, people who practiced the 4-7-8 breath saw drops in heart rate and blood pressure.[19]

- **Sighing breath.** Inhale through your nose, filling your lungs, then exhale forcefully through your mouth with a sigh. This "physiological sigh" has been shown to decrease anxiety and tension. Be sure that the exhale is longer than your inhale. As an example, count in for four and out for eight.

- **Box breathing.** Inhale through your nose for a count of four. Hold your breath for a count of four. Exhale through your mouth for a count of four. Then hold your breath again for a count of four. (If you want to shorten or elongate this exercise, you can do box breathing with any count.)[20]

- **Diaphragmatic breathing.** Also known as belly breathing, this technique invites you to breathe deeply into your abdomen rather than your chest. To try it, place one hand on your chest and the other on your belly. As you inhale slowly through your nose, aim to have only your bottom hand rise—your belly expanding like a balloon. Then exhale gently through your mouth, letting your belly fall. In one study, people who practiced diaphragmatic breathing after a stressful event had lower heart rates, reduced stress hormones, and less inflammation.[21]

If tuning into your breath feels a little too intense, you're not alone—and you're not out of options. One study found that when people paired mindfulness with sensory experiences—such as calming scents, gentle visuals, and even seeing their own heartbeat reflected back to them—they felt more relaxed and connected.[22] It turns out, weaving in your senses can make mindfulness feel a lot more approachable. So if sitting in stillness or focusing just on your breath doesn't feel quite right, try lighting a candle you love, listening to soft music, or even watching the trees outside while you breathe. There's no one right way to do this.

Get Good Sleep

Lisa, a forty-three-year-old graphic designer and single mother of two tweens, appeared to have everything under control. She manages a team at work, juggles parenting responsibilities, and keeps up with the endless demands of daily life. But when night falls, a different reality sets in.

As soon as she lies down, her body resists rest. Her mind races with all the anxieties of the day that she can't quiet, and just as she begins to drift off, a sudden jolt pulls her back into wakefulness, her heart pounding as if she's in danger. On the rare nights she does manage to sleep, nightmares invade her rest, leaving her shaken and drenched in sweat. For Lisa, sleep isn't a refuge—it's a battleground.

Lisa's struggles with sleep aren't just random insomnia; they stem from a history of childhood trauma. She endured repeated sexual abuse as a child, and while she's done the hard work of therapy and healing, her body still reacts as if danger is just around the corner. The hypervigilance she developed in childhood to survive is still showing up decades later, robbing her of the deep, restorative rest she needs.

Lisa isn't alone. Sleep issues are extremely common in trauma survivors, especially those with PTSD. In fact, studies show that 70 to 91 percent of individuals with PTSD struggle with falling or staying asleep.[23] While it's easy to assume that sleep disturbances are just another symptom of PTSD or depression, research suggests otherwise—sleep disturbances aren't just a consequence of trauma, they are also a "predisposing, precipitating, and perpetuating factor for PTSD."[24]

**Sleep isn't just rest—it's regulation.
When trauma interrupts sleep, it also
disrupts the body's ability to cope.**

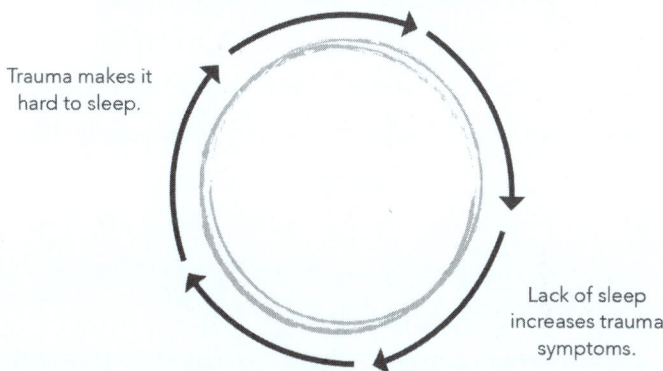

Trauma makes it hard to sleep.

Lack of sleep increases trauma symptoms.

Trauma and sleep are deeply intertwined. When trauma keeps the body in a state of hypervigilance, rest becomes difficult, and the lack of sleep only worsens trauma symptoms, reinforcing the cycle.

When sleep becomes disrupted, it can create a vicious cycle—unrested nights lead to heightened stress, increased emotional reactivity, and a body that remains stuck in survival mode. Over time, this ongoing sleep disturbance can make it even harder to regulate emotions, process trauma, and find safety in your nervous system. If you've experienced trauma, you may notice certain patterns in your sleep that reflect your nervous system's response to past threats. Do any of the following sleep challenges sound familiar?

- **Do you associate your bedroom with fear?** Your bedroom, bed, or nighttime may trigger distressing memories.

- **Are you a light sleeper, always hypervigilant about your environment?** You may wake up at the slightest sound, constantly scanning for danger.

- **Do you struggle with anxiety, rumination, or racing thoughts?** Your mind may replay past events or worry about the future, making it difficult to fall asleep.

- **Do you experience chronic pain that disrupts your sleep?** Conditions such as fibromyalgia, muscle tension, migraines, or joint pain—often exacerbated by trauma—can make getting comfortable at night diffult and disrupt sleep.

- **Do you feel a surge of energy at bedtime instead of winding down?** Your nervous system may stay in an activated survival state, keeping you wired when you need to rest.

- **Do you frequently have nightmares?** Disturbing dreams, often related to past trauma, may wake you in distress and make you fear going back to sleep.

- **Do you avoid sleep altogether?** You may stay up too late, keep the lights or TV on, or find other ways to avoid nightmares or intrusive thoughts.

- **Do you feel disconnected from reality or your body before bed?** You may fall into dorsal shutdown energy or a numb state as a protective mechanism when trying to fall asleep.

- **Do you have trouble breathing at night?** Trauma-related changes in your nervous system may contribute to sleep apnea, hyperventilation, or irregular breathing patterns.

Getting poor sleep night after night is a big inflammatory red flag. After a bad night's sleep, you feel like crap because your cells feel like crap. Research has found that insufficient sleep is linked to inflammation through a number of different mechanisms. First, sleep allows your blood pressure to drop, but when you don't get enough sleep, your blood pressure stays higher, activating inflammation within the blood vessel walls. Second, during sleep our brain takes out the garbage—the beta-amyloid protein—that is linked to brain cell damage. Without good sleep, this cleaning process is less effective, allowing the protein to build up and cause inflammation.[25] The good news? Sleep is a modifiable risk factor for inflammation, meaning there *are* steps you can take to improve sleep quality and reduce its inflammatory impact.

When a client comes to me with sleep issues, I start by looking at their nutrition—not because it's always the main cause but because it's within my scope of practice and area of expertise. Before referring them to a therapist or sleep specialist for sleep hygiene support, I want to rule out any diet or gut health factors that might be contributing to their sleep problems.

Research has shown a strong connection between sleep, metabolism, and digestion.[26] When sleep is disrupted, it can throw off metabolic processes, leading to poor dietary choices, gut imbalances, and even increased risk for conditions such as GERD, IBS, and IBD. At the same time, these conditions can make it harder to sleep by causing bloating, acid reflux, pain, and discomfort at night.

In my practice, I screen for the following nutrition-related risk factors when working with someone who has trouble sleeping:

- **Are you eating foods that support sleep?** Foods rich in tryptophan, magnesium, zinc, and B vitamins help regulate serotonin and melatonin—key hormones for sleep. Missing out on protein, whole grains, or nutrient-dense foods means you may be lacking the building blocks for good sleep.

- **Are you consuming stimulants that interfere with sleep?** Caffeine (in coffee, tea, soda, and chocolate) can linger in the system for up to ten hours, making it harder to fall and stay asleep. Alcohol, while it may seem relaxing, actually disrupts REM sleep, leading to fragmented sleep cycles.

- **Are you eating too close to bedtime?** Large or heavy meals before bed can lead to reflux, bloating, or discomfort, which makes it harder to relax. I often see this in clients who skip meals during the day and then eat a big dinner late at night.

- **Do you have gut symptoms?** Conditions such as lactose intolerance, IBS, and GERD can cause bloating, cramps, heartburn, and digestive upset, which can wake someone up multiple times during the night. If you frequently experience gut symptoms, it's worth working with a nutrition provider or gastroenterologist to get relief.

- **Is your blood sugar stable throughout the night?** Blood sugar fluctuations can disrupt sleep, causing nighttime awakenings, restlessness, or early morning wakeups. I often work with clients to balance their blood sugar by adjusting meal timing, incorporating a fat-, protein-, or fiber-rich snack before bed.

Struggling with Sleep? It Might Be Time to Get Tested

Did you know that lack of sleep affects every body system—from hormones and metabolism to your gut and heart health? If you're struggling with sleep, it's worth digging deeper. The good news is that many sleep tests can now be done at home, so you might not need an overnight stay at a sleep center to

get answers. Talk to your primary care doctor about your options and ask if a referral for at-home sleep testing makes sense
for you.

Beyond nutrition, good sleep hygiene is critical to improve
sleep quality, but it's important to approach these changes with self-
compassion. Sometimes, what's considered "good sleep hygiene" can
conflict with what your nervous system needs to feel safe. For example, a completely dark and quiet room may be ideal for sleep, but
if that makes you feel on edge due to past experiences, forcing yourself into it right away might not be helpful. The goal isn't to rigidly
follow every rule but to experiment and see what helps you feel more
rested. If you're not ready for certain changes yet, that's okay—this
is a process, not a pass-or-fail test. Work toward these practices at
your own pace, and remember that you're not failing if you're not
"there" yet.

Here are some sleep hygiene practices to consider:

- **Establish a consistent sleep schedule.** Go to bed and wake
  up at the same time every day, even on weekends. This regu-
  larity will help train your nervous system to expect predictable patterns, which will relieve stress and anxiety.
- **Create a bedtime routine.** Set the intention to tell your body
  sleep is coming by winding down thirty to sixty minutes
  before bed with calming activities such as reading, taking a
  warm bath, or doing a little stretching. I also love to drink tea
  before I go to bed, but I have to be cautious that the amount
  I'm drinking isn't going to wake me up in the middle of the
  night because I have to use the bathroom.
- **Optimize your sleep environment.** Keep your bedroom
  dark, quiet, and cool. If a dark or quiet bedroom feels

triggering for you, it's worth discussing with a therapist. Use blackout curtains or an eye mask to block out light.

- **Use a guided meditation for sleep.** There are lots of great apps out there that offer guided meditations specifically for sleep, and you can also find free options online. Even a short practice before bed can help quiet your mind and ease you into rest.[27]

- **Get those curtains open early in the day.** This will help regulate your circadian rhythm. One of my interns asked a client to try getting sunlight in the morning, and the client's response was, "Do you want me to wander around the cul-de-sac in my nightgown?" You can if the urge strikes, but I suspect the intern was just trying to see if the client could open the shades and maybe take a walk around the block—in proper clothing, of course—before going to work.

Avoid intense exercise, doomscrolling on your phone, or stressful conversations right before bed. If possible, schedule therapy sessions earlier in the day rather than in the evening—talking about trauma can activate your nervous system, making it harder to fall and stay asleep. Digital devices like phones, tablets, and televisions emit blue light that can suppress melatonin, delay sleep onset, and stress your nervous system, making it harder to fall and stay asleep. Too much screen time in the evenings has also been linked to disrupted circadian rhythms, poor sleep quality, and increased anxiety.[28] If you're noticing that your phone is keeping you up at night, consider turning off notifications or switching to a wind-down mode an hour before bed.

Sleep Looks Different for Everyone

Just like your food preferences and nutrition needs, your sleep style is personal. What works for your friend might not work for you—and that's okay. The key is finding what helps *you* get the rest you need.

If trauma-related hypervigilance or triggers make it hard to sleep, here are some specific options that may help:

- **See a therapist who specializes in cognitive-behavioral therapy for insomnia (CBT-I).** In the recent European Insomnia Guideline,[29] CBT-I received the strongest level of endorsement as a sleep intervention specific to trauma.

- **Consider using a weighted blanket.** A recent study found weighted blankets safe and effective for insomnia. One caveat: don't use a weighted blanket to sleep if you have obstructive sleep apnea or if it sends neuroceptive messages of panic.[30]

- **If you have obstructive sleep apnea, use a CPAP machine.** In one study of veterans with subclinical PTSD, those who didn't use CPAP had increased PTSD symptoms.[31]

- **Shift the layout of your bedroom.** Do this if the current setup feels unsafe or triggering.

You may also want to include trauma-sensitive mindfulness practices such as yoga nidra. Yoga nidra is a gentle, accessible practice that can help bridge the gap between the challenges of sleep disturbances and the restorative rest your body craves. While it alone won't solve your sleep problems, it's a powerful addition to other sleep hygiene practices and therapeutic approaches. Unlike traditional yoga, there are no physical poses involved—just lie down or recline comfortably while listening to a guide.

Yoga nidra works by systematically relaxing the body and mind, guiding you through different levels of awareness. It helps you activate a regulated state and has been shown to reduce trauma symptoms in veterans.[32]

Use a Sauna Regularly

I will be the first to admit that this is my *favorite* anti-inflammatory approach, although access can be a real challenge. Sure, it has been shown in multiple studies to lessen inflammation, lower your cholesterol and blood pressure, and reduce the risk of cardiovascular disease by mimicking the physiological responses produced by moderate-intensity physical activities such as walking, but I just think it feels awesome.[33]

Sauna bathing is often safe, even for those who have cardiovascular disease such as a heart attack or stroke, but it is important to check with your physician if you've been diagnosed with one of those conditions prior to use. Also, more is not necessarily better. Start slow, with five-to-ten-minute sessions, and make sure you hydrate before and after.

Go to the Dentist

Seeing the dentist might not be the most exciting way to lower inflammation, but it's one of the most effective. Poor oral health can quietly fuel low-grade, chronic inflammation, contributing to issues such as depression, anxiety, and other chronic health problems.

Here's why: Harmful toxins called lipopolysaccharides (LPS) can sneak through weakened gum tissue, a process researchers call "leaky mouth." Once LPS gets past your gums, it triggers your immune system to ramp up inflammation, spreading those inflammatory signals throughout your body.

Studies have found real connections here. One showed that people with periodontitis (serious gum disease) had a higher risk of developing depression later on. Another study linked poor oral health to both anxiety and depression in teens.[34, 35]

The good news? Regular dental visits can lower LPS levels, help rebuild a healthy oral microbiome, and reduce the inflammatory messages traveling from your mouth to your brain and body. It's a simple step that can have a big ripple effect on your health.

If you're dealing with anxiety, depression, or trauma, something as seemingly simple as brushing your teeth can be a challenge, not to mention actually going to the dentist. If getting dental care has been a struggle, you're not the only one. The majority of adults in the United States have some level of dental anxiety, ranging from mild to severe.[36]

If making an appointment for a cleaning feels too challenging today, that's okay. Reach out to the dentist in advance of the appointment. Your anxiety is almost certainly something the dentist has dealt with before. I've had clients find it very helpful to call the office in advance of their appointment and talk to the front office staff about their anxiety. They may have options you've never considered, including sedation options, scheduling early in the day to avoid rumination, or even a therapy dog! My dentist even has TVs on the ceilings of every room and subscribes to every TV subscription service that exists. Do whatever oral hygiene is accessible to you now, and consider some of these options when you do schedule an appointment:

- Schedule a simple checkup or cleaning first. Knowing it's a low-pressure appointment can decrease the risk of overwhelm.

- Bring a friend or a family member and have them sit with you.
- Agree on a hand signal with the dentist that you can make if you need a break.

Move Your Body

If you love to exercise and have a solid routine in place, feel free to move to the next section.

Still reading? I got you. I've noticed that people who have experienced trauma seem to have two very common reactions to exercise. First, there are people for whom exercise is healing, and regular exercise is part of what helps them reduce anxiety.[37] In the other group are those who see exercise as an overwhelming task, a Mt. Everest–size step that feels insurmountable. If this is you, you're not alone. In one study of people with PTSD, 30 percent of study participants were involved in exercise before the onset of PTSD, but only 6 percent exercised afterward due to the depression they were experiencing.[38] I've also noticed that some people avoid exercise because it creates uncomfortable body sensations, such as an increased heart rate or shortness of breath, which can be triggering.

Why Gentle Movement Helps the Body Let Go

Did you know that movement can help release stored stress or trauma from the body? Research shows that our fascia—the connective tissue that surrounds muscles and organs—can actually hold onto tension and trauma over time. This highlights something many people feel but can't always explain: The body remembers. Movement, especially gentle or mindful forms such as stretching, yoga, or somatic exercises, can be a powerful way to help the body let go of what it's been holding.[39]

But for many people, the challenge isn't with the body sensations of exercise or depression keeping them sedentary; it's that exercise doesn't always feel great right away. Maybe getting to the gym feels impossible. Or, even if you manage to finish a workout, you might feel . . . nothing. It can be really hard to add in exercise when you aren't getting the immediate benefits. Instead of getting caught up in the idea that you need to feel amazing immediately, it might be more helpful to reframe why you're trying to move your body in the first place. Perhaps you choose to take a walk because you feel stuck with something you're working on. Or you stretch because you feel a sore back from sitting all day.

Movement can also be a practice; it doesn't have to be exercise. If you hate the gym, you have my full permission to not go to the gym. If high-intensity workouts leave you feeling more drained than energized, it's time to find a gentler, more supportive option such as walking or yoga. In fact, excessive exercise has been found to contribute to inflammation, at least in part by increasing intestinal permeability. Endurance athletes have a higher-than-average incidence of GI disorders and show more pro-inflammatory cytokines such as CRP.[40]

Instead, clients have often found that slower, repetitive movements that come with walking, jogging, swimming, or participating in gentle yoga flow classes can really support safe neuroception. Yoga actually has been studied for PTSD with some really positive results. Yoga appears to increase activity in the parasympathetic nervous system (rest and digest) as well as GABA activity (antianxiety), which help bring you out of survival states.[41] One of the other great benefits of yoga, as well as any type of exercise, is an increase in brain-derived neurotrophic factor (BDNF), which is a chemical that will promote the growth and development of new neurons in your brain, helping with depression, anxiety, and PTSD.[42]

I was chatting with a friend recently who felt stuck because she was told by her doctor that she should exercise for a full hour every day. When we looked at her schedule, between work and shuttling the kids to after-school activities, it was clear that this wasn't realistic! So, we started brainstorming some fun alternatives to get her moving. One idea she came up with was starting a morning dance party to get her kids pumped up for the day. Just three minutes of dancing turned out to make a huge difference; it made their mornings more fun and helped her sneak in some movement without changing her whole routine.

The cool thing is that once you start believing you can do something positive for your health, it gets easier to find little ways to move throughout the day. Instead of stressing about following strict exercise rules, you can try things that feel good and don't feel like punishment. And who knows? They might help reduce inflammation and support your healing from trauma. It's all about finding what works for you and making it a part of your life in a way that feels good.

What sounds interesting? Here are some suggestions.

- **Reframe movement as a "stuck solver."** Instead of seeing exercise as a task, reframe it as a tool. Take a walk when you're feeling stuck or uninspired. It's not about the workout; it's about clearing your head.
- **Incorporate fun.** Make movement something you enjoy. Try a quick dance party with your favorite song or playful activities with your kids or pets. Movement doesn't need to feel like exercise; it can just be fun.
- **Focus on relief.** When you feel stiff or achy from sitting too long, think of stretching as a way to relieve discomfort, not as something you "have to do" for fitness. Stretching can be soothing and relaxing.

- **Break it into small bites.** You don't need to carve out a full hour to exercise. Sneak in movement with small tasks—such as walking around while on a phone call, taking the stairs instead of the elevator, or doing squats while you stir your spaghetti sauce. Bonus points if you take a walk after a meal to aid your digestion and help regulate your blood sugar.
- **Rethink the definition of "exercise."** Movement doesn't have to be structured or planned. Gardening, cleaning, or even fidgeting counts! Anytime you get your body moving, it's a win.
- **Use movement to improve mood.** If you're feeling anxious or stressed, think of movement as a way to shift your emotional state. A gentle walk, stretching, or shaking out tension can help calm your mind.
- **Try child's pose.** Okay, technically this isn't "movement," but it can be a powerful reset. If your body is in a survival state, curling into a safe, supported position like child's pose may help your nervous system begin to settle. That sense of groundedness can create just enough safety to make movement feel possible afterward. Sometimes, stillness is what helps us get moving again.

Ultimately, listen to your body. Movement can be a way to connect with your nervous system needs. Tune into what your body needs—whether it's rest, gentle stretching, or more energetic movement—without judgment or pressure.

Increase Your Intake of Anti-Inflammatory Foods

One of the most modifiable ways to combat inflammation is through food—specifically, by increasing your intake of polyphenols and other anti-inflammatory compounds.

Polyphenols are powerful plant-based antioxidants found in foods such as berries, dark chocolate, green tea, and colorful vegetables. They help neutralize free radicals—unstable molecules that contribute to oxidative stress, a major driver of inflammation. By reducing oxidative stress, polyphenols support immune function, protect brain health, and help regulate inflammatory pathways. Think of them as tiny bodyguards, shielding your cells from damage and keeping inflammation in check.

What Is Metabolic Psychiatry?

Metabolic psychiatry is an emerging field that explores how your body's energy systems influence your mental health. It asks a powerful question: What if symptoms such as anxiety, depression, or brain fog are not just psychological but also metabolic?

Your brain is one of the most energy-demanding organs in your body. It relies on a steady, efficient supply of fuel to regulate mood, focus, sleep, and emotional resilience.

But when your metabolism is out of balance—because of inflammation, blood sugar instability, mitochondrial dysfunction, or chronic stress—your brain struggles to keep up.

That's where metabolic psychiatry comes in. It focuses on the connection among:

- Mitochondria (the part of the cell that makes energy)
- Inflammation and oxidative stress
- Insulin resistance and blood sugar swings

Metabolic psychiatry is still growing, but it's opening new doors for understanding how we heal—not just from trauma, but from the inside out.

The need for more anti-inflammatory, polyphenol-rich foods can show up in both mental and physical symptoms, and if you're reading this book, I'm pretty sure you could use some extra anti-inflammatories. Systemic inflammation is one of the most common metabolic impacts of psychological trauma, meaning that if you've experienced trauma, there's a good chance your body has, is, or will deal with effects of chronic inflammation. Mentally, this might look like brain fog, sluggishness, or a sense of being easily overwhelmed, making it harder to focus and regulate emotions. Physically, it can manifest as joint pain, frequent colds, skin irritation, or lingering fatigue that doesn't seem to improve with rest.

Anti-Inflammatory and Polyphenol-Rich Foods to Add to Your Diet

- **Berries.** Think blueberries, strawberries, and raspberries. These little guys are packed with antioxidants that fight inflammation. You can toss them in your morning yogurt, blend them into a smoothie, or sprinkle them over oatmeal for a tasty boost.

- **Fatty fish.** Okay, I totally acknowledge fish may not be your go-to. That's fine, just move on to the next thing. But consider that if you love Caesar salad, the dressing for which is made from anchovies, maybe try some anchovy pasta with garlic and parsley. You'll thank me later!

- **Leafy greens.** Spinach, kale, and Swiss chard are not only good for you but also help fight inflammation. Toss some in your smoothies, salads, or omelets, or try my absolute favorite way to eat greens: Sauté beet greens with a bit of garlic and olive oil. So good!

- **Nuts.** Walnuts and almonds are healthy snacks packed with good fats and antioxidants. Just a small handful makes a difference! They're great on their own or as a topping on cereal.

- **Olive oil.** Extra virgin olive oil is an anti-inflammatory gem. I use it in salad dressings, drizzle it over roasted veggies,

and even bake with it instead of butter. I've heard that some
people drink olive oil shots!

- **Turmeric.** This spice is like a golden treasure for inflammation thanks to its component curcumin. Sprinkle it on
roasted veggies, mix it into soups, or even add a little to your
smoothies or mix into scrambled eggs.

The key here is to take it slow and experiment. Instead of trying
to cram all these foods into your meals at once, pick one or two that
sound good to you and try them out over the next week. Maybe you
start your day with a berry smoothie or switch to olive oil in your
baking. Little changes can add up!

Tackling inflammation may feel like a monumental challenge,
but as we've explored in this chapter, you don't have to tackle everything at once to make meaningful progress. The good news? You
already have many tools at your disposal. Whether it's prioritizing
sleep, spending time in nature, building connections, practicing
gentle movement, or simply adding a handful of berries to your
breakfast, each step you take sends a message of safety to your body.

And just like inflammation can have a cumulative effect on your
health, so can these positive changes. Over time, the small wins add
up—your neuroception starts to shift, your body feels safer, and your
mind begins to calm.

CHAPTER 8

That Gut Feeling? It's Your Nervous System Talking

Disaster pants aren't a good look on anyone.

—Tessa O'Toole, MS, CNS, LDN, NBC-HWC

Jan was a fifty-five-year-old woman on a mission. She wanted to successfully transition to her new job and to lessen the unremitting, unpredictable symptoms of diarrhea that had flared since she started the position. She'd recently left a long-term job as the pastor at a church she loved because she felt the need for a new challenge. Now, she was exploring her options and chose to fill in temporarily at another church that was between pastors. Her new placement was really tough. The church's congregation had asked the previous pastor to leave, and when Jan arrived there was a ton of conflict and not a lot of trust. To make matters more difficult, Jan also had a two-hour commute each way, and she would often stay over at a church-owned apartment most nights.

Prior to this new role, Jan had infrequent gut symptoms, experiencing occasional reflux and bloating once a month after she ate too much spicy food. These gut symptoms were so infrequent that she never bothered to share them with her doctor, and self-treated by taking an antacid. Now, however, Jan was dealing with reflux nearly every time she ate and also had bowel urgency and diarrhea after eating, resulting in her feeling scared to eat in case she wasn't able to make it to a bathroom in time. Disaster pants, indeed. As you can imagine, eating with congregants is a pretty common part of the job, and Jan really worried that she was offending people due to her inability to eat without experiencing symptoms.

New Patterns Are Possible: Healing the Gut-Brain Connection

If you live with IBS or another disorder of gut-brain interaction (DGBI), it's easy to feel like your body is working against you. Here's a powerful reframe: Your nervous system adapted this way for a reason. But here's the good news: What was once adaptive doesn't have to be permanent. Thanks to neuroplasticity, the brain and nervous system can change. With the right support—like safe connection, mindful movement, nervous system regulation, and nourishing food—your body can learn new patterns.[1]

Jan was experiencing a special type of neuroception that I like to call "gut feelings," meaning her feelings of anxiety and overwhelm were expressing themselves through her gut. And in turn, those gut feelings were increasing her anxiety and causing her to worry every time she left the house. It became a feedback loop, where her anxiety would cause more gut symptoms, and then the gut symptoms would cause more anxiety, again and again.

Gut Feelings Feedback Loop

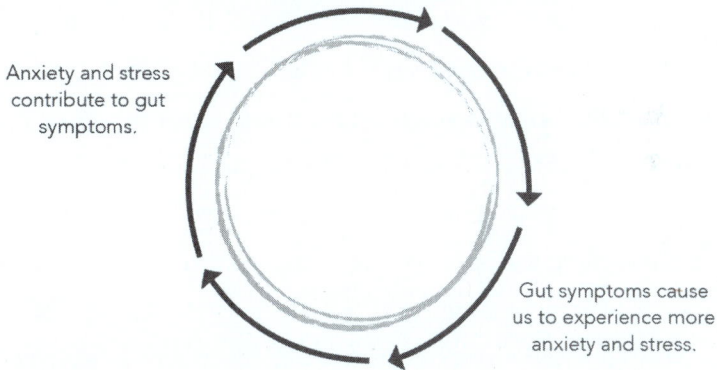

Anxiety and stress contribute to gut symptoms.

Gut symptoms cause us to experience more anxiety and stress.

Anxiety and stress activate the gut, leading to symptoms such as cramping, bloating, and urgency. These symptoms, in turn, reinforce the sense that something is wrong, increasing anxiety and making the gut even more reactive.

I'd love to say that Jan was able to completely eliminate her symptoms without changing any of the stressors in her job. Jan *did* lessen the frequency of reflux and bowel urgency to about twice a day with the diet and supplement recommendations provided. However, she had a near *complete* resolution of symptoms within a week after her placement at this church ended. Suddenly, she was back to zero bowel urgency and only experienced reflux when she ate too much spicy food. That's the power of gut feelings!

Trauma's Impact on the Gut

If you've ever had a "gut feeling" during a stressful situation, you've experienced the gut-brain connection in action. These gut feelings may cause your brain to signal the release of stress hormones such as cortisol and adrenaline, resulting in additional gut symptoms. Back and forth on the merry-go-round we go. If you're experiencing stress or trauma, the gut-brain connection can become dysregulated, leading to real physical symptoms.

So how does this work? The gut and brain are deeply connected through a complex communication network that allows them to constantly influence each other. They "talk" in several ways, but one of the most important is via the vagus nerve—the same nerve central to polyvagal theory. This long, winding nerve extends from the brainstem down to the intestines, acting as a superhighway between the brain and gut. It plays a key role in regulating digestion, stress responses, and emotional states, helping the body determine whether it is safe to rest and digest or whether it needs to stay on high alert. This two-way communication means that our digestive health and mental well-being are tightly connected—unlike in Las Vegas, what happens in the gut doesn't stay in the gut.

Trauma, abuse, and even intense stress set us up for gut disease. A meta-analysis of over 648,000 people found that those with PTSD are 2.8 times more likely to develop IBS than those without PTSD, highlighting how trauma can disrupt the gut-brain axis.[2]

Adverse childhood experiences (ACEs) significantly increase the likelihood of developing IBS and other DGBIs. In fact, each additional ACE raises the risk of being diagnosed with a DGBI.[3] A meta-analysis of twenty-three studies found a strong link between sexual abuse and functional gastrointestinal disorders such as IBS, underscoring the deep connection between trauma and gut health.[4]

Community-wide trauma can also contribute to digestive dysfunction. Following the 2018 Japan floods, disaster victims were 128 percent more likely to receive IBS prescriptions, and those without a prior IBS diagnosis were twice as likely to develop it compared to unaffected individuals.[5] This suggests that even acute environmental trauma can disrupt the gut-brain axis.

The Rome Foundation reports that between 30 percent and 56 percent of patients with functional GI disorders such as IBS report a history of trauma—including physical, emotional, or sexual abuse. These rates are significantly higher than those found in the general population, further highlighting how sensitive our gut is to our lived experience.

Trauma also worsens outcomes in inflammatory bowel disease (IBD). Among those with IBD, people who had experienced interpersonal trauma, such as domestic violence, were more likely to report severe symptoms. In nearly half the study participants, the severity of their disease was linked directly to how much trauma they had endured and how hopeless or overwhelmed they felt.[6]

Psychological stressors are also strongly associated with peptic ulcer disease (PUD). In a large population-based study of over 14,000 adults, those experiencing high levels of stress, depression, or suicidal thoughts were significantly more likely to have PUD—even when controlling for smoking, alcohol use, and chronic illness. The study found a dose-response relationship: The greater the "dose" of psychological stressors present, the greater the risk of developing ulcers in "response."[7]

As you can see, trauma isn't something that affects only mental health—it can directly impact digestion, gut function, and even the microbiome (the collection of bacteria in the gut). When we experience trauma, we shift from ventral regulation to sympathetic activation or dorsal shutdown. This shift limits the vagus nerve's ability to regulate digestion. Chronic activation of the stress response enforces the gut's experience of a survival state.

Story follows state. This is a key concept in polyvagal theory, and it means that the story your brain is telling you about what's happening—how you interpret a sensation, experience, or symptom—is shaped by the state your nervous system is in. Your nervous system sets the tone, and your brain fills in the story.

When you're in a regulated ventral state, your body feels safe. So when your digestive system engages normally with food, your brain interprets gut sensations as neutral. A little bloating after a meal might just be "oh, I'm full." A gurgle might be "my stomach is doing its job."

But when you're in a survival state—whether that's sympathetic activation or dorsal shutdown—your nervous system perceives the world as unsafe. In this state, normal digestive sensations can be interpreted as threatening. A small cramp may feel alarming. Bloating can feel like something is seriously wrong. The brain starts telling a story of danger, discomfort, or urgency—because the nervous system is sending signals of threat, even if the actual gut symptom is benign.

This is how DGBIs such as IBS develop or intensify. DGBIs are often described as "functional" because they don't have clear structural or biochemical changes; in other words, you can't see them when you scope, you can't identify them on a blood test. But that doesn't mean the symptoms aren't real. They're very real. They're just rooted in how the nervous system and gut are communicating—often in a way that amplifies pain and urgency. In the rest of this chapter, we'll focus specifically on IBS, as it is so prevalent in people who have experienced trauma.

Disorders of Gut-Brain Interaction

Just because your lab tests and colonoscopy look "normal" doesn't mean your symptoms aren't real.

〜 Irritable Bowel Syndrome (IBS)
〜 Functional Dyspepsia
〜 Functional Abdominal Pain Syndrome (FAPS)
〜 Functional Constipation
〜 Functional Diarrhea
〜 Functional Bloating
〜 Functional Rectal Pain Syndrome
〜〜Functional Nausea and Vomiting
〜 Functional Heartburn
〜〜Gastroparesis (Functional)

Disorders of gut-brain interaction (DGBIs) such as IBS and functional dyspepsia occur when communication between the gut and brain becomes disrupted, creating symptoms without visible structural changes.

A gastro-focused health psychologist I know once described IBS as a "software problem" rather than a "hardware problem," which I think is a really helpful way to understand it. Unlike conditions such as IBD, where there is clear structural damage to the intestines, IBS and other DGBIs are more about how the gut is functioning and communicating with the brain rather than something physically broken. It's a problem with the programming, not the structure—the gut and brain are miscommunicating, leading to symptoms such as pain, bloating, and unpredictable digestion. In this case, the miscommunication is that the gut thinks it is in a survival state.

How Stress, Trauma, and Infection Disrupt the Gut-Brain Connection

DGBIs such as IBS are real conditions that involve changes

in how the body functions—not visible damage, but miscommunication between the brain and gut. Trauma can play a role in
developing IBS, but it's not the only factor. For some people, it
starts after a bad gastrointestinal infection. In those cases, the
immune system tries to protect the body but ends up keeping
the gut stuck in a reactive state.[8]

Chronic stress makes this even harder. Stress doesn't just
live in the mind—it impacts the gut microbiome, weakens immune defenses, fuels inflammation, and affects mental health.
These disruptions don't happen in isolation; they feed off one
another, creating a feedback loop that keeps the body out of
balance.[9]

The good news? Understanding this connection is the first
step toward interrupting the cycle and helping your gut find its
way back to ventral regulation.

Objectively, the body and gut are safe. There's no acute infection,
food poisoning, or physical injury. But subjectively, the enteric nervous system in the gut doesn't feel safe.

Over time, stress can alter how the immune system responds and
how inflammation is regulated. Instead of resolving, these changes
can deepen existing imbalances and increase the risk for illness—
especially in sensitive systems such as the gut and nervous system.

There are, of course, cases where something *is* really off in the
gut. Conditions such as IBD, celiac disease, GERD, gallbladder diseases, diverticular disease, and peptic ulcers have clear structural,
inflammatory, or infectious causes. There are specific medical nutrition therapy approaches used with these conditions, and if you are
struggling with a non-DGBI disease, I'd recommend you see a CNS
or RD who specializes in gut nutrition.

Bottom-Up Versus Top-Down Approaches to Gut Regulation

So how do we work to provide the gut signs of safety when it has become dysregulated? One of the best ways is to use a bottom-up approach that encourages the body to talk to the brain. Bottom-up approaches such as yoga, breathwork, progressive muscle relaxation and nutrition help bring the autonomic nervous system into regulation without us having to cognitively process the trauma directly. Sure, you have to think about putting your body into a yoga pose, and think about what you'll eat for dinner, but you don't have to consciously make the yoga twist stimulate your vagus nerve or tell the blueberries to help reduce oxidative stress.

Remember, most of the communication between the body and brain—about 80 percent—actually travels from the body to the brain, not the other way around. Only about 20 percent goes from the brain down to the body. This means your brain is constantly listening to signals from your body about how safe, stressed, or balanced things feel. It's a powerful reminder that to support healing, we need to work with both the body and the mind, not just one or the other.

In contrast, with top-down approaches, you focus on changing your thought patterns, processing your feelings, and working to better understand why you believe the things you do. CBT uses a lot of top-down processing to help people change negative thought patterns that contribute to distress. The hope is that changing or reframing the thought will help you change your emotional response and behavior. "Name it to tame it" is a great therapy phrase that reflects the top-down approach of verbal processing.

Most therapy includes elements of both top-down and bottom-up approaches. The same thing applies to the practice of nutrition. When I see a client, I'm definitely helping them reframe their thoughts about food and nutrition (a top-down approach), but at the same time, I ask a ton of questions about how it feels in their body when we make shifts, and we select a nutrition approach that will bring more ventral regulation to the body (a bottom-up approach). In the next chapter, we'll talk about different foods and supplements that send messages of safety to your brain and body through a bottom-up approach.

Bottom-up Approaches Don't Require Talking About Trauma to Start Healing from It

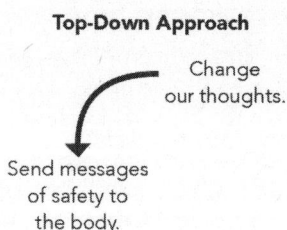

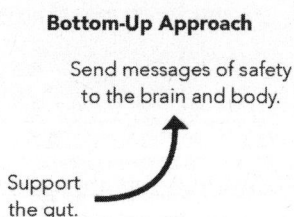

Top-Down Approach

Change our thoughts.

Send messages of safety to the body.

Bottom-Up Approach

Send messages of safety to the brain and body.

Support the gut.

Nutrition is a bottom-up approach that can change how safe your gut, brain, and nervous system feel.

But beyond food changes, there is another evidence-based way to support healing in the gut: using gut-directed hypnotherapy and imagery. This approach uses guided relaxation and focused attention to create a calm state where therapeutic suggestions can reframe the brain's interpretation of gut sensations, reducing symptoms such as bloating, pain, and irregular bowel habits. There are even some studies that indicate that gut-directed hypnotherapy can lessen the inflammatory cytokine load of IBD.[10]

You might be familiar with hypnosis for entertainment purposes —those stage shows, movies, or depictions of mind control that make it seem like hypnosis is some kind of magical power. In college I remember seeing a show where my friends were encouraged while under hypnosis to cluck like chickens! While it's entertaining, this version of hypnosis has little to do with its clinical application. Clinical hypnosis is a medically supported, research-backed approach that can address a variety of health concerns. For example, there are over thirty years of solid research demonstrating its effectiveness for gastrointestinal issues.

In contrast with entertainment hypnosis, according to Ali Navidi, a licensed clinical psychologist who specializes in gut-directed hypnotherapy, clinical hypnosis involves teaching people how to deliberately enter a self-controlled trance state and use it therapeutically to address specific challenges. Trance is a natural state of attention that we all experience daily, often without even realizing it. If you've ever driven home from work on autopilot, suddenly realizing you've arrived in your driveway without consciously remembering every turn you made, you've been in a trance state. Athletes often describe a similar experience while playing their sport. They get so caught up in the game, they might not even notice a scrape or bruise until it's all over. That kind of deep focus lets the brain zero in on what matters most in the moment and tune out anything less urgent—such as a little pain or discomfort. It's a kind of natural tunnel vision, where the mind narrows in and everything else fades into the background.

Staying Safe During Gut-Directed Hypnotherapy

If you have a history of trauma—especially trauma that's led to dissociation, numbing, or feeling frozen—it's important to approach gut-directed hypnotherapy with intention and support. Hypnotherapy invites deep focus and relaxation, which can be incredibly healing—but for some trauma survivors, it can also feel too unstructured or unsafe, especially if your nervous system is used to spending time in shutdown and disconnection. If dissociation has been part of your experience, you are not alone, and this doesn't mean hypnotherapy is off-limits. But it does mean you should talk with your therapist first. Together, you can assess whether gut-directed hypnotherapy feels like the right fit and whether there are ways to adapt it so your body and brain stay regulated.[11]

In clinical hypnosis, one of the most powerful aspects of trance is how it taps into the brain's built-in ability to focus. People can zero in on certain sensations while tuning out others—like turning down the volume on pain or anxiety. This focused attention helps many folks manage discomfort in a way that feels doable.

Pain management is one of the most well-known ways this principle gets used. Through hypnosis, people can shift their focus in a way that makes pain feel less intense—or they can think about it differently altogether. Someone dealing with chronic pain, for instance, might imagine a dial they can mentally turn down, giving them a greater sense of control over what they're feeling. Believe it or not, this type of approach was used as early as 1927 by researchers trying to treat IBS-like symptoms (they called it spastic esophagus and mucous colitis).[12] One of the most-cited researchers in the modern age studying gut-directed hypnotherapy is Olafur Palsson, a psychologist who developed a series of seven hypnotherapy-based scripts for IBS called the North Carolina Protocol. These scripts were meant to be used in session with a provider and include language such as the following:

> Imagine relaxing inside a warm, safe, comfortable mountain cabin like this; nothing can disturb your comfort. The thick walls protect you from all discomfort. Even though the storm is howling outside, you can barely notice it in the safe comfort of the log cabin. In the same way, you are protected more and more every day from pain and discomfort in your stomach and bowels. You are becoming less and less sensitive to discomfort or pain until nothing can upset or irritate your intestines anymore.[13]

Response rates vary by the clinical trial, but generally they are very high, from 53 to 94 percent.[14] Other hypnotherapy protocols such as the Manchester Approach and the Bremner Method have also been studied. Research has shown that gut-directed hypnotherapy is as effective as a low-FODMAP diet, making it a great alternative for people with IBS who want to avoid having to eliminate foods from their diet. It's been successfully used with adults and children, with people who have severe IBS, and with people who have a hard time being hypnotized. It's also been found successful in people who didn't respond well to other treatments.[15]

One big challenge is that it can be hard to find a therapist who specializes in gut-directed hypnotherapy. Often, you can find these providers working in the outpatient gastroenterology department (you read that right) of large hospitals. Depending on the hospital, you may need to see a gastroenterologist in the department to get access to their psychologist. I've also referred many clients to GI

Psychology, a group therapy practice that sees clients in all US states. Visit them at www.gipsychology.com.

Unlike gut-directed hypnotherapy, which requires a practitioner to help you through it, gut-directed imagery is a guided meditation you can listen to on your phone. Just like with gut-directed hypnotherapy, gut-directed imagery encourages the mind to "reframe" its interpretation of gut sensations, reducing anxiety and fostering positive associations with digestion. For example, an app might guide you to imagine your gut as a calm, flowing river, where everything moves smoothly and comfortably. By repeatedly engaging in these exercises, the brain can rewire its responses to gut signals, sending calming messages to the body instead of alarm signals.

I do love how easy gut-directed imagery apps are to use. Tools such as Happy Inside have helped many clients reduce GI symptoms.

How Does This All Work?

We don't actually know yet! It doesn't appear that gut-directed hypnotherapy actually changes anything in the gut microbiome, suggesting that hypnosis improves IBS through shifting the neuroception of the gut by calming the autonomic nervous system.[16] Gut-directed approaches also combat the feeling of powerlessness that so many people with IBS have, which can have a profound psychological impact.

For years, I was guilty of underestimating the power of gut-directed mind-body approaches. After carefully honing a specialized diet and supplement regimen to keep my IBD calm, I just got used to having to restrict certain foods. Within eight weeks of starting individualized gut-directed hypnotherapy with a psychologist, I added back five foods I wasn't able to previously eat and had an 80 percent reduction in my GI urgency and diarrhea. Of course, when I get stressed, my GI symptoms will often come back, but a single session with my therapist often cuts symptoms off completely. These days, I don't introduce gut-directed mind-body options as the last recommendation to my clients; I encourage them to get access to it as soon as reasonably possible.

CHAPTER 9

Your Gut May Have Trouble Maintaining Good Boundaries; Support It

> Setting boundaries is a form of self-love.
>
> —Shefali Dang

You've likely heard about why maintaining boundaries in relationships—both personal and professional—is important to your mental well-being. The same can be said about gut boundaries, which you probably didn't even know existed until now. The gut lining is one of our most essential boundary systems, acting as a protective barrier between the external environment and our internal organs. This lining, composed of a single layer of cells, stretches across the small and large intestines and is supported by a layer of mucus, tight junctions, and immune cells. Its job is to maintain selective permeability, meaning it allows the absorption of essential nutrients such as vitamins, minerals, and amino acids while preventing harmful substances such as pathogens, toxins, and undigested food particles from entering the bloodstream.

When these boundaries are intact, you're more likely to experience strong digestion, better nutrient absorption, a calm immune system, and more balanced energy and mood. But when they're compromised, the result can be increased intestinal permeability (often called "leaky gut"), which may contribute to symptoms such as food sensitivities, fatigue, bloating, brain fog, or inflammation throughout the body.

To achieve this delicate balance of allowing some things in while keeping others out, the gut lining relies on tightly regulated processes. The tight junctions between the cells act like gatekeepers, opening and closing in response to physiological cues to let in nutrients and keep harmful substances out. However, this highly controlled system can be disrupted by different factors:

- Chronic inflammation from inflammatory bowel diseases such as Crohn's and ulcerative colitis
- Diets low in fiber
- High alcohol consumption
- Excessive exercise
- Chronic survival state activation due to stress and trauma

Maintaining gut boundaries supports not just your digestion but your whole-body health—including immune resilience, mental clarity, and emotional regulation. But just like in our emotional lives, when those boundaries are worn thin or pushed too hard for too long, they can lose their ability to protect us.

When the integrity of the gut lining is compromised, a condition known as *intestinal permeability*—often referred to as "leaky gut"—can develop. I prefer to use the phrase *gut boundaries*, as I feel like this resonates more with mental health—because in many ways, what happens in the gut *is* deeply mental and emotional.

When your gut's protective boundaries weaken, harmful particles such as LPS—toxins from certain bacteria—can slip through the gut lining and enter your bloodstream. Once inside, they send a distress signal to your immune system, triggering the release of inflammatory cytokines.

But this inflammation doesn't stay in the gut. Those cytokines can travel through your blood and cross into the brain, activating the brain's immune cells, called microglia. Normally, microglia help protect and repair brain tissue. But when they stay activated too long, they can cause damage—disrupting how brain cells communicate, altering mood circuits, and even leading to structural changes in the brain.

Neuroinflammation also affects brain chemistry. It can lower dopamine and serotonin (important for mood and motivation) while raising glutamate and reducing GABA (which increases feelings of stress and anxiety).

And here's where the cycle deepens: Once the brain becomes inflamed, it can send stress signals back to the gut—weakening the gut lining even further and throwing off the balance of your microbiome. This creates a feedback loop where gut problems fuel brain inflammation, and brain inflammation makes gut issues worse.

In short, what starts in the gut doesn't stay there. It ripples outward, influencing how you feel, think, and respond to the world around you.

Once we understand how critical gut boundaries are—and what can happen when they break down—the next question is: What can we do about it?

There are two main strategies I use to help restore and support gut boundaries. Each has its place, and depending on your story, different strategies may be more appropriate for your nervous system and what your body needs most. Let's walk through them.

Consider the Amount of Potentially Inflammatory Food You Eat

This is probably the most popular method discussed on social media and arguably the one that gets oversimplified the most. While it might seem like the obvious first step—just eat fewer inflammatory foods and more anti-inflammatory ones—it's not usually my go-to starting point. For many people, especially those living with trauma, it's just not that simple.

You see, your gut may be inflamed not because you're eating the "wrong" foods but because your nervous system has been stuck in survival mode. Trauma alters the way the gut-brain axis functions. So even if your plate looks "perfect" by nutritional standards, your gut may still be sending out distress signals: reacting to foods not because of their content but because your system is hypervigilant.

When I first started my nutrition practice more than ten years ago, elimination diets were the standard approach. Someone would come in feeling foggy, fatigued, and bloated, and we'd take them off a long list of potential trigger foods. And it *worked*. People felt better—for a while.

But then something would happen.

Over time the relief would fade. And they'd start reacting to more foods—the ones they had kept in. So we'd eliminate those too. And so the cycle would continue, shrinking their food world further and further until every bite felt like a threat. Eventually, the lack of dietary diversity would become a danger signal itself, leaving the gut even more reactive and the nervous system more on edge.

That's why I no longer recommend elimination diets as a one-size-fits-all solution. If you have a clear, repeatable reaction to a specific food, removing it temporarily can be helpful. But that decision should be made with the guidance of a qualified nutrition provider—someone who can not only help you identify what to avoid but, more importantly, help you reintroduce foods and rebuild trust in your gut again.

Decrease the Body's Reaction to the "Scary Stuff" (Such as LPS)

Even if we can't control the body's reaction to everything that enters the gut, we can work to regulate how our body responds. That's where the concept of vagal tone comes in. When your vagal tone is strong—that is, when your nervous system is flexible and resilient and you spend time in ventral regulation—your body can better tolerate the presence of things such as LPS without launching a massive inflammatory response. That means fewer symptoms of inflammation, even if the gut lining isn't perfect.

But there's another key piece to this puzzle: digestion itself. One of the simplest ways to reduce inflammatory triggers in the first place is to make sure your food is being fully digested. Why? Because your gut will react to what you don't digest. (I feel like there is a therapy metaphor in there somewhere!) What do I mean by this? One of my clients has lactose intolerance, and if he eats two pieces of pizza, he's fine. But three pieces? His wife wants to kick him out to sleep in a tent in the backyard due to the farts. Now, your symptoms may not be as obvious as his—unless you also have lactose intolerance and eat lots of dairy. But it is really common for people to have less-than-optimal digestion or an eating hygiene that sets them up for symptoms hours later.

Digestion isn't just about breaking down food into nutrients; it's also about ensuring that what passes through the gut doesn't linger, ferment, or cause inflammation. Under normal circumstances, our digestive system is well equipped to handle most foods we consume, breaking them down into usable nutrients. However, stress, poor eating habits, suboptimal stomach acid levels, and low digestive enzyme levels can all interfere with this process, leaving partially digested food to travel through the intestines. When digestion isn't working efficiently, the gut is more likely to react to these unprocessed particles as if they were threats, which can lead to inflammation and disrupt gut boundaries. As I described earlier, this immune response doesn't just stay in the gut; it can affect our mental health, increasing feelings of anxiety and contributing to the cycle of "gut feelings" that reinforce stress.

Believe it or not, you actually start digesting your food far before it reaches your stomach. Even the smell or sight of food starts saliva forming in the mouth, cueing the digestive system that food is about to arrive. Ideally, we are regulated when this happens. Our digestive systems don't work as well (or at all) when we're in a survival state of sympathetic activation or shutdown. I'm going to list some common practices I use with clients, but I want to invite you to listen to your own nervous system here. If the suggestions I'm making don't feel safe for you, follow your own wisdom.

Create a Calm and Relaxed Eating Environment

The state your nervous system is in when you eat can make a huge difference in how well you digest your food. Eating in a regulated state sends a signal of safety to your gut, helping your digestion work the way it's supposed to. But when you're stressed, rushed, or overwhelmed, your body shifts its energy away from digestion— because in survival mode, it thinks there are bigger emergencies to deal with. That's when you're more likely to experience things such as bloating, discomfort, or feeling like food just sits in your stomach. Whenever you can, try to create a little bit of connection or calm before eating. Whether that's sharing a meal with someone you care about or simply taking a few deep breaths before you dig in, small moments of ventral regulation can really make a difference.

Of course, eating in a perfectly regulated state isn't always realistic. Sometimes you're grabbing a bite between meetings, managing a toddler meltdown at dinner, or eating in the car on your way to work. Life is messy—and that's okay. The goal isn't 100 percent compliance or perfection. It's about slowly tipping the balance, spending more meals in ventral regulation and fewer in a stress state.

Eat Slowly and Savor Your Food

Recently, my colleague Tessa O'Toole told me a story about one of her clients. This fourteen-year-old boy had recently gotten his braces tightened. The pain he experienced as his teeth adjusted made chewing difficult. When she asked how he was managing, he told her, "I'm just swallowing my food whole!" My mom-brain was pretty scared at this choice, but thankfully nothing dire happened. When he later mentioned having some "interesting poops," Tessa knew exactly why. By eating slowly and savoring your food, you reduce the workload on your stomach and intestines, allowing them to digest food more efficiently and absorb nutrients better. Eating slowly also sends "rest and digest" messages of safety to your brain, anchoring you in ventral regulation.

How Mindful Eating Supports Your Gut

Mindful eating plays a key role in healthy digestion and overall well-being. When we slow down, chew our food well, and eat in a calm state, we help our bodies digest and absorb nutrients more easily and reduce the effects of stress on the body. Protein is especially tricky to digest when we're stressed or not eating mindfully. Stress—whether emotional or physical—can affect the gut lining, throw off our gut bacteria, and lower the levels of stomach acid and enzymes needed to break food down properly. When digestion isn't working well, it can lead to bigger issues such as inflammation, immune problems, and added stress on the nervous system. Eating with awareness isn't just about food; it's a simple but powerful way to support your whole body.

Sometimes, unfortunately, we're in a rush. This is where the technique of savoring helps. In her book *Anchored*, Deb Dana describes savoring as a process that helps you lean into ventral regulation energy for a moment. As a nutrition provider, I encourage clients to savor their first bite of food. If you actually savored every bite, you'd be sitting at the table for hours. But savoring just the first bite takes less than a minute. This savoring process involves three steps:

- First, you become aware that you're about to eat food that you can savor.
- Next, you become present and appreciate that first bite.
- Finally, you give that sensation all your attention for twenty to thirty seconds.

Voilà! You've savored the first bite! You can savor with the first sip of tea or coffee, you can savor with sliced apples and cheddar cheese, and of course you can savor with ice cream. Whatever foods allow you to tune in to the present moment and give your full attention are great for this exercise.

Prioritize High-Quality Sleep

Don't worry; you haven't suddenly skipped ahead to a different chapter. Sleep plays a vital role in maintaining gut boundaries and overall digestive health. Just as dreams are a way for your brain to process life events and sort through stuff, the gut takes out its garbage when you sleep. The migrating motor complex (MMC) is a critical process where a "cleaning wave" of electrical and muscular activity happens in the gut, clearing out undigested food particles, cellular debris, and bacteria. This allows the gut lining to repair itself, ensuring that it maintains its role as a strong boundary. Poor sleep, on the other hand, can increase gut boundary issues and disrupt the balance of gut bacteria, leading to inflammation and other digestive issues.

The Circadian Rhythm of Your Microbiome

Did you know your gut has a clock too? Scientists have discovered that the gut microbiome follows a daily rhythm, just like the rest of your body. This internal clock—also known as your circadian rhythm—helps regulate important systems such as digestion, metabolism, immunity, and even your mood. When your body's rhythm is out of sync, it can affect how these systems work, and vice versa. For example, poor sleep or chronic stress can disrupt your gut, and an imbalanced gut can make it harder to sleep or feel calm.[1] The good news is that you don't need a complete life overhaul to get back in sync.

Simple, everyday habits can make a big difference. Things such as getting sunlight in the morning, sticking to a regular bedtime, and powering down screens before bed help keep your body's rhythm on track. These small shifts support your gut and, in turn, your mood, energy, and digestion.

When you prioritize these digestive hygiene habits, you create an environment where your gut can function at its best. These small but intentional shifts can strengthen the gut-brain connection, reduce stress-related digestive issues, and lay the groundwork for a healthier, more balanced digestive system.

Feeding Your Gut Boundary What It Needs to Thrive

Imagine trying to bake an apple pie without apples—impossible, right? The same principle applies to your gut. Without the right "ingredients," your gut can't produce the chemicals that help you feel calm, connected, and safe. These ingredients come in the form of specific nutrients that fuel the production of neurotransmitters and gut-healing compounds. For instance, amino acids from proteins are critical for producing serotonin, the "feel-good" chemical. Fiber from fruits, vegetables, and whole grains feeds beneficial gut bacteria, which in turn produce short-chain fatty acids that reduce inflammation and support mental health. Omega-3 fatty acids from foods such as fish and flaxseeds help regulate stress hormones and reduce systemic inflammation. Think of this as your nutrient recipe for safety—a way to give your gut exactly what it needs to produce the signals that help you feel your best. So, what food does it need to make these messages?

Fiber

Fiber is more than just roughage—it's the foundation of a well-fed microbiome, the collection of bacteria in your gut. When certain fibers reach the large intestine, they become food for your gut bacteria, which ferment them into short-chain fatty acids (SCFAs) such as butyrate, acetate, and propionate. These SCFAs help fuel the cells that line your gut, reinforce barrier function, and reduce inflammation —not only in the gut, but throughout the body, including the brain.

Why Short-Chain Fatty Acids (SCFAs) Matter

SCFAs aren't just important for gut health—they're essential for brain health too. These powerful molecules, produced when your gut bacteria ferment fiber, help maintain emotional resilience, lower inflammation, and support the gut-brain connection.

Each SCFA plays a unique role:

- Butyrate boosts brain-derived neurotrophic factor (BDNF), promotes the growth of new neurons (neurogenesis), and reduces neuroinflammation—key for mood, memory, and recovery from stress.
- Acetate strengthens the gut barrier, helps balance the immune response, and reduces inflammation linked to anxiety.
- Propionate regulates the body's stress response, supports neurotransmitter production, and plays an important role in mood regulation.[2]

When SCFA levels drop, mental health symptoms such as anxiety, depression, and brain fog can worsen. Supporting a healthy microbiome through fiber-rich foods and targeted gut therapies is one of the most powerful ways to nurture both your gut and your mind.

Butyrate is especially powerful. It helps keep the tight junctions between intestinal cells snug, protecting your bloodstream from invaders such as LPS. But its influence doesn't stop there. Butyrate also helps maintain the integrity of the blood-brain barrier and sends calming signals to the nervous system that can support mental health, improve sleep, and reduce perceived stress. In short, the more butyrate your gut can make, the more resilient you may feel—both physically and emotionally.

So, how do you make more butyrate? It starts with eating more fermentable fibers—such as those found in oats, apples, berries, root vegetables, brown rice, and legumes. Resistant starch is another powerful ally. This unique type of starch is formed when starchy foods like potatoes or rice are cooked and then cooled. The cooling process changes the starch structure, making it resistant to digestion in the small intestine and available for fermentation in the colon. (And yes, you can reheat them—resistant starch survives the warming-up process.) These resistant starches can promote better gut health, support your microbiome, and contribute to steady energy and mood regulation.

You can also get small amounts of butyrate directly from food—most notably from butter. So yes, adding butter to your steamed vegetables might actually help your gut lining, not hurt it.

That said, fiber isn't universally beneficial for everyone. For people with IBS or other forms of digestive sensitivity, some fibers—especially the fermentable ones known as FODMAPs—can be a major trigger. Foods such as garlic, onions, beans, and certain fruits may cause gas, bloating, or discomfort due to the fermentation process. And if you're dealing with slow motility or constipation, suddenly adding lots of fiber can actually make things worse.

This doesn't mean fiber is off the table—it just means you may need to get more specific. Different types of fiber interact differently with the gut:

- Soluble fiber (found in oats, citrus fruits, apples, and legumes) tends to form a gel-like substance and can help with both diarrhea and constipation.
- Insoluble fiber (in wheat bran, carrots, cabbage, and corn) adds bulk and helps move things through but can aggravate some IBS symptoms.
- Resistant starches (in cooled rice, potatoes, and green bananas) feed beneficial bacteria and promote SCFA production.

The key is slow experimentation. Try adding small amounts of different types of fiber, one at a time, and notice how your body responds. If things run more smoothly—more regular digestion, less bloating, improved mood—that's a sign your gut is saying yes. If symptoms flare, back off or shift to a different type.

In this way, fiber becomes not just a nutrient but a feedback loop. Your body will tell you what's working. Your job is to listen.

Polyphenols and Antioxidants

Eating colorful foods isn't just about making your plate Instagram worthy; it's one of the simplest ways to support your mental health. Colorful fruits and vegetables are packed with polyphenols, powerful plant compounds that act as antioxidants and anti-inflammatories. These compounds don't just help your cells stay healthy; they play a critical role in calming the gut, supporting the brain, and reducing the inflammatory effects of LPS.

When it comes to protecting the brain from inflammation, a few natural compounds have shown some pretty exciting results—at least in early studies with animals and cells. Here's a quick tour:

- **Curcumin (from turmeric).** Curcumin has been shown in animal studies to help protect memory and prevent brain inflammation triggered by LPS. Rats given curcumin didn't show the same memory problems as those that weren't.[3]
- **Resveratrol (from grapes).** This compound has powerful anti-inflammatory and antidepressant effects. In mouse studies, resveratrol helped improve memory issues caused by LPS and even reduced brain cell damage and inflammation.[4]
- **EGCG (from green tea).** Green tea's superstar antioxidant, EGCG, has been shown to calm overactive immune cells in the brain. By cutting down oxidative stress and inflammation, EGCG may help shield the brain from damage linked to toxins such as LPS.[5]
- **Lycopene (from tomatoes and watermelon).** Lycopene doesn't just make tomatoes red—it also seems to help protect the brain. In mouse studies, lycopene reduced inflammation and oxidative stress, helping prevent memory problems tied to LPS exposure.[6]
- **Hesperetin (from citrus fruits).** Found in oranges and lemons, hesperetin has shown brain-boosting benefits too. Mice that got hesperetin were much better at learning and remembering things, even after facing LPS-induced stress on the brain.[7]

Including polyphenol-rich foods such as turmeric, grapes, green tea, tomatoes, and citrus fruits in your diet may help support brain health and reduce inflammation. While the studies I mentioned looked at isolated compounds found in these foods—not the foods themselves—they offer promising clues about how everyday foods might protect against LPS-driven neuroinflammation. You don't need to load up on a bunch of supplements; simply weaving more of these whole foods into your meals can be a gentle, supportive way to nourish your brain and body.

Can What You Eat Help Ease Anxiety?

A recent study looked at how certain nutrients found in fruits, veggies, and tea—called flavonoids—might help lower anxiety. Researchers found that people who ate more flavonoids were less likely to show signs of anxiety.

Some of the most helpful flavonoids included the following:

- Naringenin (in citrus fruits)
- Genistein (in soy)
- Apigenin (in chamomile and parsley)
- Flavones and flavanones (found in many fruits and vegetables)

Even small amounts of these flavonoids seemed to make a difference. What you eat really can affect how you feel. Adding more colorful fruits, leafy greens, citrus, soy foods, and herbal teas to your diet might be a natural way to help support your mood and ease anxiety.[7]

Polyphenols also play a big role in supporting BDNF. BDNF is a protein that's crucial for neuroplasticity—the brain's ability to adapt, grow, and rewire itself—and it's also important for regulating mood. Want top-down therapy approaches, like reframing thoughts or changing how you respond to stress, to actually *stick*? Then you're going to want healthy levels of BDNF on your side. It helps your brain build new pathways and shift old patterns into ones that feel more supportive.

While it doesn't exactly fit into this chapter, I'd be remiss if I didn't also tell you that movement matters too. Brisk walking, for example, is a powerful (and simple) way to boost BDNF production, giving your brain even more ability to "refire and rewire." In fact, if you want therapies such as CBT to be more effective, supporting your BDNF levels is a smart move.

Vitamins and Minerals

Certain vitamins and minerals are essential for gut health, particularly vitamin D, zinc, and magnesium. Vitamin D helps regulate the immune system in the gut, reducing inflammation and supporting the gut's microbial balance.

Zinc plays a direct role in maintaining the gut boundary integrity, and magnesium supports relaxation and helps regulate gut motility, reducing the risk of constipation and its effects on the gut lining. You can get more vitamin D from fatty fish like salmon, fortified dairy or plant-based milk, eggs, and sunlight exposure. Zinc is found in oysters, beef, pumpkin seeds, and chickpeas. To get magnesium, you'll want to add more leafy greens like spinach and kale, as well as almonds, cashews, and whole grains.

Probiotic Foods

Probiotics are live bacteria found in fermented foods that can add beneficial strains to the gut microbiome. Certain probiotic genuses, such as *Lactobacillus* and *Bifidobacterium*, are associated with improved mood and reduced anxiety. By promoting a healthy gut microbiome, probiotic-containing foods can help send safety messages to the gut and the brain and reduce stress responses. How do they do this? Bacteria produce beneficial byproducts known as postbiotics, which significantly impact gut health and brain function. Postbiotics include SCFAs such as butyrate, acetate, and propionate that were mentioned when we discussed fiber, as well as precursors to neurotransmitters such as serotonin, dopamine, and GABA. Certain bacteria in the gut also synthesize a lot of the B vitamins we need for mental health including folate (37 percent of RDA), vitamin B12 (31 percent of RDA), and B6 (86 percent of RDA).[8]

Why Gut Type Matters for Stress and Diet

Not everyone responds to food the same way—and your gut microbiota might be why. In a study of 810 participants, researchers found that the relationship between dietary habits and stress responses depended heavily on the type of gut bacteria people had (their "enterotype").[9]

- For some people, eating certain foods frequently was linked to *lower* stress levels.
- For others, the same eating patterns were linked to *higher* stress levels.

Your gut community influences how your body and mind react to food. This could explain why dietary changes help some people more than others when it comes to managing physical or psychological symptoms. Your gut's unique fingerprint plays a bigger role than we ever realized.

One thing to note: If you choose to experiment with adding probiotic foods and you're getting uncomfortable symptoms of gas, bloating, constipation, or diarrhea after eating, you're not alone. Increased gas and bloating can occur when adding probiotic foods to the diet because they introduce new bacteria or feed existing gut bacteria, leading to increased fermentation in the gut. Some people need an adjustment period, where they gradually increase their intake of probiotic foods. If the increased gas and bloating persists, consider seeing a nutrition provider. They may be able to recommend some basic shifts in food or provide supplement ideas to lessen your symptoms.

You can also take supplements that contain probiotics, but you want to use caution to get the right strain. Probiotics that have effects on mental health are called psychobiotics, and when you pick one, you're going to want to get the specific type that has been studied for your symptoms. Probiotic names can be a bit confusing at first because they include multiple parts: the genus, species, and the strain. Each part of the name provides information about the specific bacteria and its unique characteristics. Here's how probiotic names are structured:

- Genus—the first part of the name that refers to a broad group of bacteria, such as *Lactobacillus* or *Bifidobacterium.*
- Species—the second part of the probiotic name that provides more information about the specific type of bacteria. An example would be "acidophilus" in *Lactobacillus acidophilus.*
- Strain—the third part of the name is a more specific identifier that helps you understand the unique properties or benefits of the probiotic. An example would be "GG" in *Lactobacillus rhamnosus GG,* which is a probiotic strain that is being studied to reduce PTSD symptoms in veterans.[10]

When I pick a probiotic for a client, I'm trying to match up the genus, species, *and* strain with the results that I'm looking for in the research literature. As an example, if I have a client with anxiety, I will look for products that contain *Bifidobacterium longum 1714* and *Bifidobacterium breve 1205,*[11] not just products that contain *Bifidobacterium longum* and *Bifidobacterium breve.* The strain really does matter; it indicates the specific formulation of a product that has been studied for a specific set of circumstances. Here are some formulations of psychobiotics that have been studied to support mental health:

- If you want to reduce psychological distress, consider *Lactobacillus helveticus R0052* and *Bifidobacterium longum R0175*.[12]

- If you want to lessen gut symptoms that are related to stress, consider *Lactobacillus casei Shirota*.[13]

- Want to support mood? You might want to try a combination of *Bifidobacterium bifidum W23, Bifidobacterium lactis W52, Lactobacillus acidophilus W37, Lactobacillus brevis W63, Lactobacillus casei W56, Lactobacillus salivarius W24,* and *Lactococcus lactis W19* and *W58*.[14]

I'm almost positive you are wondering how on earth you'd ever find these options. Product availability changes so frequently, I'm choosing not to provide specific brand names here. Instead, visit my website sources for a list of current psychobiotics that I recommend.

Diversify Your Diet

Dietary diversity—eating a wide range of different foods—is key to cultivating a safety-promoting microbiome. A varied diet introduces different fibers, nutrients, and compounds that feed different types of beneficial bacteria. A diverse microbiome is more stable and resilient, meaning it's better able to send messages of neuroceptive safety via the gut-brain axis, produce beneficial metabolites, and protect against gut dysbiosis. When the microbiome is diverse, it can adapt more readily to stress, reducing the impact on gut and mental health.

While it might seem overwhelming at first to increase your dietary diversity, it is possible if you know a few good tips:

- Salad bars with a mix of fresh fruits and vegetables are a boon for increasing dietary diversity. Sure, you're paying a lot per pound, but on the other hand, are you really going to go to the grocery store, buy twenty-five different foods, and cook them? If you just want to try a few bites of a new fruit or vegetable such as red cabbage, buy just a few tablespoons worth from the salad bar.

- Spice mixes are also going to be your friend. If you don't already have some on hand, explore blends from different geographic regions, as that's the best way to make sure you're getting as little overlap as possible. As an example, a blend of Italian herbs and spices is likely to include different ingredients than curry powder.

- Pick different brands or varieties of fruits and vegetables than you normally get. Sure, those two different brands of carrots look the same, but they were likely grown in different places, have different types of bacteria on them, and can be a great and easy way to add some diversity. Normally get gala apples? Give honeycrisp a try.

Repairing gut boundaries isn't about doing everything perfectly; it's about offering your body a little more safety, a little more support, day by day. Some days you'll eat mindfully. Some days you'll grab a snack in the car. It's all part of the process. What matters is the overall direction you're heading: more connection, more nourishment, more trust in your body's ability to heal. Small changes make a big difference over time. Your body—and your mind—are always listening. And they're capable of more healing than you might realize.

CHAPTER 10

Stress Shapes Your Symptoms: How to Build More Resilience

I try to take one day at a time, but sometimes several days attack me at once.

—Jennifer Yane

"I'm so stressed," Christy said as she walked into my office, plunked her purse on the floor, and sank into my couch. A forty-two-year-old director of development for a large nonprofit and mother of three young kids, Christy felt chronically underwater, but this week she seemed more tired than usual. "All three kids have had strep throat, so I'm working from home, but the house next door is being torn down. Between the sick kids inside and the banging outside, I haven't had a peaceful moment in weeks. Food has been a joke, I feel like I have zero control over what I eat, and to make it even worse, I can't even remember to take my supplements. I'm getting constant headaches, and I know my blood pressure is spiking." I knew that Christy was up against a deadline for a series of grant applications for the nonprofit she worked for, a task that required dedicated, focused attention, which these days was sorely lacking.

I'd been seeing Christy for two months, focusing on nutrition and lifestyle support for her blood pressure. Christy was hoping to avoid medication, and her doctor gave her six months to try to get her numbers down. Although Christy had great intentions to eat right and exercise while in my office, she kept hitting barrier after barrier at home. Between the kids' needs, the intense stress caused by potential budget cuts at work (hence the need for additional grants), and a husband who regularly traveled and wasn't really present when he *was* home, Christy struggled to find time to take care of herself.

I knew Christy felt embarrassed to come to session, week after week, having struggled to add more fruit and vegetables to her diet as we discussed. But after hearing the load she carried on a daily basis, I wondered whether we should focus first on nervous system regulation. "Christy," I asked, "what percent of the day do you feel like you're in a survival state?" For a long moment, she looked out the window at my bird feeder and the yellow finches eating seeds, then sighed and said, "100 percent of the time." I took a moment to let that sink in and asked, "And when was the last time you remember feeling regulated?" After another long sigh and drink of her coffee, she said, "I can't remember the last time." I wish I could say Christy was the exception, rather than the norm, of clients I see.

Stress isn't always bad. As early as 1908, psychologists Robert Yerkes and John Dodson proposed that a certain level of stress is necessary to promote performance and achievement. Go above that level, however, and performance suffers. In the 1930s, Hans Selye coined the term *eustress* to describe positive or good stress that provides optimal levels of stimulation. Present-day researcher Alia Crum builds on this foundation, showing that it's not just the stress itself but rather our perception of stress that matters. In her study *Rethinking Stress: The Role of Mindsets in Determining the Stress Response,* Crum showed participants videos that showed stress to be either enhancing (improving focus and performance) or debilitating (causing harm to health). The people that watched the "stress is enhancing" videos had better physical responses to stress. In other words, the stress response was more moderate and resolved more quickly than for the people who watched the "stress is debilitating" video.

Let's pause here for a moment. Reframing stress or shifting your mindset can be helpful—but it's not a cure-all, especially if you've lived through trauma or long-term stress. That's because stress isn't just something you *think* or *feel*—it's something your body *goes through.* It's a whole physiological experience driven by your nervous system.

Polyvagal theory reminds us that our sense of stress and safety comes not just from what we think but how our autonomic nervous system responds. If, like Christy, you've lived in a state of chronic stress, your nervous system remains on high alert, even if you are objectively safe. Instead of asking, "How can I change my mindset about stress?" I'd invite you to ask, "What does my nervous system need to feel safe?" Let's start by looking at some of the ways that your nervous system perceives stress and encourages movement to a survival state.

In an interview on the *Sounds True* podcast with Tami Simon,[1] polyvagal therapist Deb Dana said, "Neuroception is this lovely way that our nervous system is listening to what's going on. It listens through three streams of awareness. It listens inside our body to what's happening in there in our viscera, in our muscles, in our organs. It listens outside into the world around us, and that world can be the world immediately around us and then out into the larger world around us. And then also between us and other people, on a nervous-system level rather than a brain level."

Inside

As I've discussed in previous chapters, some stress comes from inside. Inflammation, stress hormones such as adrenaline and cortisol, distress signals from the gut, and nutrient depletion send neuroceptive signals of danger to your nervous system, often outside your conscious awareness. What you likely do consciously feel are the impacts of chronic illness or pain in your body, from IBS to fibromyalgia to many other diseases.

This internal stress—especially when it's chronic—can shift how your body uses the nutrients you take in. One key example is how the amino acid tryptophan is processed. Normally, tryptophan (which you get from protein-rich foods) helps produce serotonin, the neurotransmitter that supports mood and calm, and eventually melatonin, which regulates sleep. But under stress, your body reroutes tryptophan down what's called the kynurenine pathway instead.

This shift happens when the immune system is activated or when inflammation is present—conditions that often accompany chronic stress, illness, or trauma. Instead of making serotonin, the body uses an enzyme called IDO (indoleamine 2,3-dioxygenase) to convert tryptophan into kynurenine, which can then produce quinolinic acid. Quinolinic acid has been linked to neuroinflammation and excitotoxicity—it overstimulates certain brain receptors, activates the brain's immune cells (microglia), and can trigger symptoms such as anxiety, low mood, brain fog, or sleep issues.

You don't have to consciously think your way into stress for this to happen; your body perceives the signals and reacts. Gut issues, microbiome imbalances, poor digestion, and even intestinal permeability (i.e., leaky gut) can all amplify this process, pushing more tryptophan into the kynurenine pathway and away from mood-supportive serotonin.

Elevated levels of quinolinic acid have been found in people with depression, PTSD, chronic fatigue, and other conditions where inflammation and stress intersect. This is one way your body's internal signals can deeply affect your mood, energy, and resilience—without you even realizing what's happening behind the scenes.

Understanding this helps us appreciate that healing isn't just about mindset—it's about calming the body's stress biology from the inside out.

Outside

External stressors are all around us and send both visible and invisible signals of danger. For some, this includes the harsh realities of living in active war zones or regions of political instability where the nervous system is responding to real, ongoing threats. But even in places where danger isn't immediately life-threatening, loud environments, poor air quality, road rage during your commute, and even the constant jarring ping of email alerts can keep the nervous system on high alert, pushing it into survival mode.

I've been incredibly privileged to live in safe environments in my life—neighborhoods where I don't have to lock the door to take the dog out for a walk or even lock my car at night. I've never been so humbled to understand the vast impact that the environment has on the nervous system as in the summer of 2024, when a cicada brood awoke from its seventeen-year slumber and crawled out of the ground to invade my Illinois neighborhood. Now, on the surface, cicadas are benign. They don't sting or bite, they aren't poisonous, and the only damage they do is to young trees by laying too many eggs in their branches.

Many of my neighbors found them charming, eagerly awaiting each new stage of the cicada life journey. I, however, hated them. The sound was constant and deafening, sometimes topping 100 decibels, similar to a lawn mower or rock concert. Even inside our house, I could hear them from the moment the sun came up in the morning until sundown when they finally ceased their mating calls. Every single time we went outside we'd have to dodge cicadas. They would land on your clothes, your face, and even get caught in your hair. I thought they looked terrifying, with big bodies and bright red eyes, and a length of one to one and a half inches. These weren't small bugs. One summer day I was unlucky enough to close the car door just as one flew in. What resulted was a truly embarrassing moment of panic, complete with arms flailing, accidental horn honking, and multiple failed attempts to get my seat belt off and the car door open all the while the cicada was zooming around the car. I hated every single minute.

I didn't just hate the cicadas; my nervous system was actively destabilized by them. It didn't matter that objectively I was safe and the cicadas couldn't harm me. I didn't feel safe. Luckily, my nervous system was able to calm down when the cicadas died off, and I won't have to deal with them for another seventeen years. Not everyone is that lucky. Have you experienced any of these "outside" stressors to your nervous system?

- **Sensory overload.** Fluorescent lighting, loud noises, crowded public spaces, or cluttered and disorganized spaces
- **Little connection to nature.** Lack of sunlight, poor access to greenery or trees or time outside, or living in a concrete-heavy neighborhood
- **Environmental or chemical exposure.** Mold in poorly ventilated homes, toxin exposure in food and water, the Flint Michigan water crisis, and East Palestine, Ohio, train derailment
- **Natural disasters.** Los Angeles fires, Hurricanes Katrina and Harvey, and the Maui wildfires
- **Mass shootings.** Columbine High School, Virginia Tech University, Sandy Hook Elementary, Marjory Stoneman Douglass High School, and Pulse Night Club
- **Recessions and financial crises.** The dot-com crash, the subprime mortgage crisis and subsequent recession
- **Illness.** Covid pandemic, increasing rates of measles and tuberculosis

It's important to remember here that even small stressors that may not impact your friends or neighbors can have a large impact on your nervous system. Your past experiences of trauma and chronic stress have likely tuned your nervous system to identify your home away from home (a survival state) as the new normal.

How Stress Reaches Down to Your Cells

Chronic stress from trauma doesn't just affect how we feel—it can impact the entire body on a cellular level. Research shows that ongoing stress can damage our mitochondria, the tiny energy producers inside our cells. When this happens, it can trigger a chain reaction of inflammation and oxidative stress, mess with how our cells make energy, and even change how our DNA works. One important part of the brain involved in all this is the amygdala—best known for handling fear and alerting us to danger. But newer studies show it also helps regulate the immune system. When trauma keeps the amygdala on high alert, it can throw the whole system out of balance, keeping the body stuck in a state of inflammation.

In Between

Some of the most challenging stress comes from our relationships with others. Our nervous systems are built for connection—they seek out cues from the people around us to help us feel safe and understood. When we're in challenging relationships and experience repeated conflict and abuse, our nervous systems get stuck in a survival state. This relationship tension doesn't have to be "dramatic" to make an impact. It can be as "little" as a friend who talks over you when you're sharing your day, a partner who goes silent when you need support, or the parent that loves you but frequently steps over boundaries. And, of course, the relationships you have may be toxic or abusive:

- A boss who claims credit for your work
- A friend who judges you for your body shape or food choices
- A romantic partner that tells you that you're "too sensitive" or are "overreacting"
- A parent that only engages with you when they need something from you
- Anyone who hurts you physically, calls you names, or uses intimidation to control you

And it doesn't always take conflict or abuse to make an impact. Engaging regularly with dysregulated people can put our system through stress, especially if you are a highly sensitive or empathetic person. Whether the neuroceptive signals are subtle or overt, relationships like these can contribute significantly to stress, by teaching you to anticipate harm rather than connection.

What Is EMDR—and Why Do People Use It for Trauma?

EMDR stands for Eye Movement Desensitization and Reprocessing. It's a type of therapy that helps people process painful or overwhelming memories so they don't keep affecting everyday life. Instead of retelling your trauma story in detail, EMDR uses gentle, back-and-forth stimulation—like eye movements, tapping, or sounds—while a trained therapist helps you stay grounded and present.

Over thirty research studies have shown that EMDR can be effective for both adults and kids. It's often used for PTSD, anxiety, and other trauma-related symptoms. Because trauma memories can get "stuck" in the nervous system, EMDR helps the brain and body reprocess those memories so they can feel less intense—and finally stay in the past, where they belong.

If you've ever felt like your body is reacting to things that "shouldn't" be a big deal, EMDR might be a helpful way to shift that. Just make sure to work with a trauma-informed therapist trained in EMDR so you can move through the process safely and at your own pace.

Systemic oppression such as racism, ableism, fatphobia, anti-LGBTQ+ bias, and misogyny provide chronic input that you aren't safe, and the nervous system will adapt by staying in a state of hypervigilance. Your nervous system remembers when your body isn't welcome.

Each of these stress signals—inside, outside, or in between—can stretch your nervous system thin. But when they stack up, they can tip your body into survival mode without you even realizing it.

When Christy said she was stressed 100 percent of the time and food felt out of control, it wasn't just for a single reason. Christy had multiple inside, outside, and in between factors that were putting her nervous system into a survival state. *Inside*, she was experiencing hypertension along with frequent headaches, fatigue, and feeling on edge. It didn't feel possible to get the anti-inflammatory and antioxidant-rich fruit and vegetables she needed, and life was so chaotic that even taking supplements was tough. *Outside*, she experienced the jarring noise from the construction site next door, as well as the sometimes very loud noises of her children. Work also contributed to her stress, with worry that budget cuts were forthcoming if she didn't win new grants. *In between*, her relationship with her husband was not supportive, and given her busy life, she didn't have time to regularly connect with friends.

It's likely that Christy would have the ability and nervous system resources to cope with any one of these stressors, but all of them collectively were more than her system had the ability to navigate without turning to a survival state. For Christy, trying to "do more" only pushed her nervous system more into overwhelm. She didn't need more information on what to eat or another supplement to attempt to take. She needed to experience more moments of safety that didn't increase her workload.

This is where understanding heart rate variability (HRV) becomes very helpful. HRV is the microvariation in time between each heartbeat. We often imagine our hearts beating like a metronome, with a steady, regular beat with no variation between the intervals.

In actuality, that lack of variation in a heart rate suggests a nervous system that is very stressed.

In contrast, microvariations between the heartbeats means your body is able to adapt and respond to your environment. Instead of a metronome, we want an orchestra conductor that is able to speed up or slow down the tempo in response to the moment, drawing out a swell when needed and softening when it's time to rest. That's what healthy HRV looks like. It's not about being perfectly calm all the time; it's about having the capacity to shift states fluidly, to rise to meet a challenge and then return to calm when the moment has passed. HRV reflects that internal flexibility. It shows us whether your nervous system is stuck in one gear or able to move between nervous system states.

What About All Those Vagus Nerve Hacks?

If you've spent time online lately, you've probably seen a flood of advice about "vagus nerve hacks"—cold plunges, humming, gargling, deep breathing, splashing your face with cold water, or even foot massages. Some of these practices *can* support vagus nerve function, but not all of them work the same way for everyone.

Stimulating the vagus may improve digestion, mood, and your body's ability to handle stress. That said, there's a lot of individuality in how your body responds. What calms your neighbor might feel agitating to you—and that's not a failure. It's feedback. There's no one-size-fits-all solution. The best "hack" is learning how *your* nervous system responds and finding ways to make friends with it. What helps you shift into a state of safety? What practices feel regulating?

When your HRV is high, it's a signal that ventral regulation is active—that your body feels secure enough to rest, digest, and relate. When stress becomes chronic or traumatic, the nervous system starts to rely more heavily on survival states: sympathetic activation or dorsal shutdown. In these states, HRV typically drops. Your system gets stuck in defense mode, and the rhythm of your heart reflects that lack of flexibility.

Many people think that if they just try harder they can force their way into regulation. But HRV doesn't work that way. It's influenced by your body's real-time sense of safety, and it can actually impact how regulated your eating is. In one study, teens with lower HRV had significantly higher food cravings and lack of control of eating.[2] Another study found that the heart rhythm patterns of people who struggle with loss of control around food may reflect how well they can manage emotions. The people who felt out of control with food or frequently overate had lower HRV at rest—a sign that their nervous system may be less flexible or less able to calm down after stress.[3]

Many diseases are associated with low HRV, including hypertension, type 2 diabetes, IBS, chronic fatigue syndrome (ME/CFS), depression, generalized anxiety disorder and panic disorder, PTSD, sleep disorders, and autoimmune conditions including FM.

For Christy, although she had already started to focus on food, it made sense to shift our work toward nervous system regulation and increased heart rate variability. We started with breath. Christy put sticky notes on her bathroom mirror to remind her to take a few breaths with the exhale longer than the inhale. When she had time, she'd search for "breathing pace six breaths per minute" on YouTube and align her breath to the videos. When the kids recovered from their illness and she was able to go back into the office, she'd use her in-bound commute to play her favorite music and sing along in the car. The commute home was dedicated to listening to a funny podcast and was no longer filled with last-minute calls to team members. And even though she'd hardly used her rocking chair since her kids were babies, she started using it for a few minutes before bed every night because she found the rhythm soothing.

Before long, it became easier for her to remember what safety felt like and to stay in that state for longer periods of time. As her nervous system remembered safety, she monitored her smart watch and slowly saw her HRV begin to rise. After a couple months, food didn't feel nearly as out of control, and Christy had enough emotional bandwidth to begin to include frozen, microwaveable vegetable packets with dinner every night, and eventually she was also able to meal prep simple vegetable, protein, and grain bowls for work. When she eventually made it back to her physician, her blood pressure was noticeably down, and the physician told her to "keep up the good work."

I firmly believe that, like Christy, you can increase your HRV without purchasing anything. You can focus on breathwork, physical activity, sleep, and spending time in nature as discussed in Chapter 7. You can also explore any of the food approaches listed in Chapter 5.

If, however, your nervous system likes data to validate your progress and help you feel safe, it is also possible to use biofeedback tools, apps, and wearables to monitor and improve HRV. These tools help monitor beat-to-beat intervals between your heartbeats and interpret your autonomic flexibility in real time.

HeartMath Inner Balance

HeartMath was the first HRV tool I was introduced to years ago, and it remains my go-to resource for many people learning to regulate their nervous system. The HeartMath Inner Balance system uses a small ear-clip sensor that connects to an app, providing real-time feedback on your heart rate variability. What makes it powerful isn't just the data—it's the way it teaches you to sync up your breath, emotions, and heart rhythm through a practice they call "coherence."

The app guides you through slow, steady breathing and helps you shift into a state of gratitude, appreciation, or calm focus. One of the features I love most is that the app uses sound to indicate where you are in your coherence range—meaning you don't even have to look at your phone. I've used it while watching my kid at karate, sitting in the car, or even walking—letting the sound gently guide my nervous system without needing a screen. I also recommend HeartMath for commuters. Just put the ear-clip sensor on one ear and an earbud in the other, and no one will realize you're learning to regulate while on the subway! With regular use over time, you'll increase your ability to return to ventral regulation more quickly when you're stressed.

Smart watches and smart rings also offer the ability to track HRV. Before buying a new tool, you may want to investigate whether you currently have access to an HRV monitor.

However, while HRV can be a powerful window into our internal nervous system state, it can cause people to be a little obsessive—especially when you watch it constantly. HRV fluctuates naturally over the course of a day due to a variety of factors including your sleep, hydration, stress level, and even the weather. A low-HRV day doesn't mean that you've failed or you aren't making progress; it's just information telling you that your nervous system invites gentleness.

Rather than using HRV data to criticize yourself, think of it as a pattern tracker. When you look at days that had high HRV, do you notice any regular patterns? Were those days you were able to wake up later, had the time to eat regularly, or remembered to breathe deeply? What could you take away from that experience to put in your self-care tool kit for the future?

The Heart of the Matter: How the Vagus Nerve Connects Body and Mind

The vagus nerve connects directly to the heart, which helps explain why improving HRV has such a powerful effect on both body and mind. In fact, scientists now talk about a microbiota-gut-brain-heart axis—a reminder of how beautifully interconnected our systems really are.

The good news? There are several ways you can support your HRV and boost nervous system regulation—such as managing stress, practicing deep breathing, eating nourishing foods, getting good sleep, and moving your body regularly.[4]

Likewise, on the days that your HRV was lower, did you have a huge assignment due or a tough conversation with your boss, or were you just so busy that you didn't have time to eat anything that wasn't available in the vending machine? That's okay! Looking back, are there any tools that you wish you had access to during the day that might have helped?

When Christy came into my office overwhelmed and unsure where to begin, her story reflected what so many people feel but often keep quiet: Modern life is too much for their nervous system to handle. And yet, through small, consistent shifts—breathing with intention, making space for joy, finding moments of ventral regulation even in the middle of chaos—her body began to remember what safety felt like.

HRV is just one way to track that return. Whether you're drawn to breathwork, nature, food, movement, or technology, the most important thing is that the tools you choose feel supportive rather than stressful. This work isn't about perfection—it's about building a relationship with your nervous system—one that says, "I'm listening. I'm here. I've got you."

That's the real lesson here. Ventral regulation isn't something we force. It's something we gently return to. Again and again.

You don't have to do it all at once. And you don't have to do it alone. Small steps, anchored in safety, can reshape your entire experience of stress and open the door to healing, connection, and greater vitality. Just like it did for Christy.

PART III

Building Approachable and Sustainable Nutrition Tool Kits

As you prepare to dive into these final chapters, I want to take a moment to reflect on the journey we've taken so far. Throughout these pages, you've explored how food is more than just fuel—it's deeply intertwined with your nervous system, emotions, and sense of safety. You've learned how your body's responses to food are influenced not only by the nutrients you consume but also by your mindset, environment, and nervous system state. Now, as we near the conclusion, it's time to put these ideas into action and craft a framework for moving forward.

To build these tools, we need to revisit the concept of *pendulation*, the natural movement of your nervous system between states of ventral regulation and survival. Just as pendulation allows us to move through challenging states with resilience, your relationship with food must also adapt to the ups and downs of life. To support this, you'll build two essential tool kits:

- **The Survival Nutrition Tool Kit** will guide you through moments of overwhelm or dysregulation. This is about finding simple, approachable strategies to meet your needs when everything feels too hard, reminding you that feeding yourself is always an act of care.

- **The Ventral Regulation Nutrition Tool Kit** will help you maintain balance and nourishment when life feels steady and connected. It's a chance to lean into joy and cultivate supportive habits that sustain your well-being over the long term.

As you read, I encourage you to let go of the idea that you must get everything "right" when it comes to food. Instead, focus on building a relationship with eating that feels intuitive, supportive, and adaptable to wherever you are.

The beauty of these tool kits lies in their flexibility. On some days, your Ventral Regulation Nutrition Tool Kit will feel second nature as you savor meals and explore new ways to nourish yourself. On others, your Survival Nutrition Tool Kit will remind you that eating frozen meals and snacks while watching your favorite show are not only okay but necessary. Both paths are acts of care and both are part of the journey toward ventral regulation and resilience.

By embracing this approach, you're giving yourself permission to eat in a way that is responsive to your nervous system, supporting not just your physical health but your emotional and psychological well-being too. So, let's get started building your next chapter.

CHAPTER 11

Building Your Survival Nutrition Tool Kit

Caring for myself is not self-indulgence. It is self-preservation, and that is an act of political warfare.

–Audre Lorde

"Name it to tame it" is therapist speak for the practice of naming and labeling emotions as a way to regulate them. In this chapter, we'll name what survival states look like in your life. We'll explore how your world shifts when you're in a survival state and see how your story about food follows from that survival state.

As you work through this exercise, keep in mind that we all have a "home away from home"—a nervous system state we tend to land in more often when things feel stressful or overwhelming. For some, it is sympathetic activation, which is marked by urgency, anxiety, and action. For others, it might be dorsal shutdown, marked by collapse, withdrawal, or numbness. You may find one state easier to describe than the others—that's completely okay. Just do your best.

To complete this exercise, grab a blank piece of paper and draw a simple chart like the one shown here. Draw one vertical line down the center of the page to divide it into two columns. Label the left column **sympathetic activation** and write the following prompts under it, leaving space to answer each one:

- I know I'm in this state because . . .
- Food is . . .
- My adaptive and protective responses to food are . . .
- Some unintended ripple effects are . . .
- Three words that describe my approach to food in this state are . . .

If you'd like a ready-to-use template, you can download it directly from my website: www.megbowmannutrition.com/resources.

What's Cooking in Your Nervous System?

Sympathetic Activation

I know I'm in this state because	
Food is	
My adaptive and protective responses to food are	
Some ripple effects are	
Three words that describe my approach to food in this state are	

Understanding how your nervous system shapes your food behaviors is a powerful step toward healing. This reflection helps you name how sympathetic activation shows up in your relationship with food. By identifying patterns in this state, you can respond with more self-compassion and choice.

Understanding Activation

Start by imagining or remembering a moment when you felt sympathetic activation energy in your system. Remember, there is no trauma Olympics; you don't need to remember the worst trauma you've ever experienced for this exercise to be successful. You might think about the last time a customer yelled at you at work or the day you forgot to send your kid's field trip permission slip to school.

Next, tune in to your experience during that moment: Did you feel your heart racing, your muscles tensing, or your mind spinning? Did the room get hot, did your cheeks redden, or did you feel so much restless energy you had trouble staying still? Now, keeping those feelings in mind, start filling out the middle section of the page. When you're experiencing sympathetic activation energy:

I know I'm in this state because . . .

You might notice that everything feels urgent, like there's no time to slow down or catch up. You might feel wired—restless, impatient, and easily frustrated. Some people describe feeling like they're bracing for something bad to happen, even if they can't point to a clear reason why. These are all ways your nervous system lets you know that sympathetic activation energy is in charge. In sympathetic activation energy, you might write the following:

- "I think I'm falling behind."
- "I am barely holding it together."
- "I start seeing other people as obstacles that prevent me from finishing my work."
- "I start clenching my jaw or grinding my teeth without realizing it."
- "I talk faster and louder than I normally do."

Food is . . .

When you're in an activated state, food often shifts from a simple daily act to something more complicated. It might feel like food is just another task you don't have time for or like food is fuel you need to get through the chaos of the day. Sometimes food becomes a reward for surviving the stress. Other times, it feels overwhelming—just one more decision you don't have the energy to make. For many, food becomes a source of temporary relief or escape, something that soothes the relentless hum of urgency, even if only for a few minutes. When you're feeling sympathetic activation energy, you might write the following:

- "Food is so hard to manage."
- "Food is the only break I get."
- "Food is something I don't have time for."
- "Food is out of control and impossible to resist."
- "Food sits in my stomach like a brick."

My adaptive and protective responses to food are . . .

In this state, your nervous system is trying to protect you the best way it knows how. You might find yourself grabbing whatever's quickest, even if it's not what you truly want. Some people skip meals altogether because their bodies feel too revved up to even register hunger. Others find themselves rigidly controlling every bite, trying to create a sense of order when everything else feels chaotic. Emotional or mindless eating can also be a response, especially when stress peaks and your system reaches for anything to ground itself. Sometimes people wait until the world feels quieter—late at night—to finally eat in a way that feels safer or less exposed. You might write the following:

- "My adaptive and protective response to food is eating whatever's fastest, even if it's not good for me physically."

- "My adaptive and protective response to food is skipping meals because I feel too overwhelmed to eat."
- "My adaptive and protective response to food is to track every bite I eat so I feel in control."
- "My adaptive and protective response to food is to eat in secret so no one can judge me."
- "My adaptive and protective response to food is to binge at night when the world finally feels quiet."

Some ripple effects are . . .

While these protective strategies are rooted in survival, they often come with side effects. You might find yourself crashing hard in the afternoon because you didn't eat enough energy earlier. You might end up overeating at night and feeling physically uncomfortable. Some people notice they stay wired and anxious after relying on caffeine instead of food for energy. Others feel guilt or shame about how they handled food during stressful periods. Over time, these patterns can leave you feeling more exhausted, both physically and emotionally, than you realized—and often still not truly nourished. An example of an unintended ripple effect might be:

- "I feel totally drained because I skipped meals and now have zero energy."
- "I get shaky and irritable by late afternoon because I haven't eaten enough all day."
- "I overeat at night after not eating much earlier, and then I feel so full I can't sleep."
- "I rely on carbs to get through the day, and then I crash hard an hour later."
- "I drink coffee instead of eating and then feel wired and anxious."

We'll come back to the final prompt—choosing three words that describe your approach to food in this state—at the end of the chapter, after you've had time to explore and reflect.

This exercise was eye-opening for Sam, a forty-year-old accountant and single mom to a ten-year-old son. Sam had grown up in a household where food was tightly controlled—portions were monitored, treats were earned, and there was always a running commentary about weight and "eating right." As an adult, she was trying to break that cycle. She wanted food to feel nourishing, not loaded with guilt or rules, especially now that she was raising a child of her own.

But every year, tax season pulled her into old patterns. It hit like a tidal wave, and Sam would show up to our sessions looking completely worn thin—tired eyes, shoulders tight, clutching a lukewarm coffee at two in the afternoon. She described this time of year as "living in a pressure cooker." The endless stack of tax returns meant long days at the office, followed by evenings at home helping her son with math homework. "I feel like I'm sprinting all day and never get to stop," she told me.

We did the What's Cooking in Your Nervous System exercise together during one of her toughest weeks in March. I asked her to think about a recent moment that captured her activated energy. She paused, then said, "Wednesday night. My son was crying about his homework, I still had ten returns to finish, and I hadn't eaten anything but vending machine snacks since breakfast. I felt like I was going to explode."

I invited her to pause and take a breath, then write down her answers to the prompts:

I know I'm in this state because . . .

"Everything feels urgent. I can't sit still. My heart races, my chest feels tight, and I snap at small things without meaning to."

Food is . . .

"Food is just another thing I don't have time for. It's a distraction from what I have to get done."

My adaptive and protective responses to food are . . .

"I skip meals because eating feels like wasting time. I drink coffee to push through. I grab whatever's closest, usually junk, because it's fast."

Some ripple effects are . . .

"I crash hard by late afternoon. I get shaky and irritable. I feel ashamed for not eating better, and the coffee wrecks my stomach."

As we discussed her answers, Sam realized that when she was falling behind at work, she felt like she had zero permission to eat. She noticed how deeply the old message—that food had to be earned—was still wired into her body's response to stress. She also commented that she'd be heartbroken if her son learned to treat himself the same way. For Sam, this realization was the first step in beginning to shift the cycle and offer herself more compassion—and nourishment—during survival seasons.

Understanding Dorsal Shutdown

Now that you've explored your experience in sympathetic activation energy, we're going to explore what it feels like to go numb and shut down. You might not even recognize it right away because it can feel like dissociation, fogginess, or like the world is just too much.

To begin, take a moment to remember a time—not the worst time, just a moment—when you felt like you had too little energy. Maybe you were so emotionally exhausted you didn't return a friend's text, or you found yourself zoning out in front of the TV while your to-do list sat untouched. Maybe it was the feeling of hiding under the covers, not because you were sleepy but because the day just felt too much to face.

Once a flavor of that memory is within reach, see if you can tune in to what your body felt like. Were you exhausted, slumped, or slow? Did your thoughts feel far away, or did your mind go blank? Maybe you felt invisible—or wished you could be.

Now, take another piece of paper, and complete the following prompts as shown here:

What's Cooking in Your Nervous System?

Dorsal Shutdown

I know I'm in this state because _____

Food is _____

My adaptive and protective responses to food are _____

Some ripple effects are _____

Three words that describe my approach to food in this state are _____

This reflection activity helps you recognize how dorsal shutdown shapes your relationship with food. By naming your experience, you gain awareness of how exhaustion, collapse, or disconnection influences your eating habits.

I know I'm in this state because . . .

When you're in dorsal shutdown—disconnected, collapsed, or numbed—the world can feel far away, like it's happening behind a thick pane of glass. You might notice feeling exhausted, heavy, or like you're moving underwater. You might write the following:

- "I am numb."
- "I feel invisible."

- "I am too tired to try."
- "I am a burden."
- "I am not really here."
- "It's hard to lift my head or make eye contact."
- "It's hard to form words or find what I want to say."

Food is . . .

When you're in a dorsal shutdown state, food can lose its usual meaning or feel strangely disconnected. It might seem like food is irrelevant—something you can't muster up the energy to care about. Sometimes food feels dull and tasteless, almost like an afterthought. Other times, food becomes a way to feel *something* when everything else feels numb. You might find yourself eating mechanically, not really tasting anything, or feeling indifferent to whether you eat at all. For many, food in dorsal shutdown isn't about managing stress or getting through the day—it's about trying to bridge the deep sense of disconnection from body and life. When you're feeling dorsal shutdown energy, you might write the following:

- "Food is pointless."
- "Food is something I do without thinking."
- "Food is a way to feel something, even if it's not what I need."
- "Food is tasteless, but I eat anyway."
- "Food is the only thing that reaches me when nothing else can."

My adaptive and protective responses to food are . . .

When you're in a dorsal shutdown state, your body and brain may be moving through the day on autopilot, disconnected from hunger, taste, or routine. Maybe you find yourself not eating at all— meals come and go without notice, and the idea of preparing food feels impossible. Or maybe you go through the motions, eating in front of a screen or grabbing whatever's easiest, not really tasting anything but not able to stop. Some people swing between extremes: not eating all day because there's no energy or drive, then numbing out with whatever's around at night. When you're feeling dorsal shutdown energy, you might write the following:

- "My adaptive and protective response to food is not eating because I can't find the energy to care."
- "My adaptive and protective response to food is eating whatever's easiest without noticing how much or how often."
- "My adaptive and protective response to food is eating mindlessly in front of the TV because it feels safer to stay numb."
- "My adaptive and protective response to food is ignoring hunger until it becomes overwhelming and urgent."
- "My adaptive and protective response to food is turning to food late at night when loneliness or emptiness feels the strongest."

The ripple effects are . . .

These protective patterns can create ripple effects. You might wake up feeling bloated or uncomfortable because you ate more than your body could easily handle. You might notice your energy is even lower the next day because you didn't nourish yourself in a way your body needed. Digestion often suffers too; people in dorsal shutdown often report feeling constipated, nauseous, or experiencing swings between extremes. Emotionally, dorsal shutdown eating patterns can reinforce feelings of disconnection, isolation, and frustration. You might notice these ripple effects:

- "I feel guilty and uncomfortably full because I didn't realize how much I was eating."
- "I have zero energy because I've barely eaten all day."
- "When I eat this way, my digestion is off—I'm either bloated or constipated."

Here's an example of how Jessi, a twenty-eight-year-old student getting her master's degree in social work, explored her experience of dorsal shutdown through this exercise.

Jessi came into our session feeling numb. "I'm just so tired," she said, staring down at her hands. She had just turned in a big project and was juggling internship hours, classes, and a part-time job. But it wasn't just exhaustion that bothered her. As we started talking, she admitted, "I don't feel like myself. I'm going through the motions, and I just can't stop eating."

We talked about the nervous system's response to burnout and what it feels like to be in dorsal shutdown mode.

I asked Jessi to answer these prompts:

I'm in this state because . . .

"The world feels far away, muffled, and too much. I am numb, alone, and feel like I don't matter. I can't find the energy to move or care about anything."

Food is . . .

"Food is something I reach for to fill the emptiness. It's not about hunger—it's the only thing I feel connected to in that moment."

My adaptive and protective responses to food are . . .

"I skip meals without noticing because I'm too disconnected to feel hunger. Then at night, I overeat because my body is desperate for something—anything—to wake me up. I eat quickly, standing up, not really tasting it."

Some ripple effects are . . .

"My stomach hurts in the morning, and I don't feel hungry again until late afternoon. Then the cycle starts over. It makes it harder to focus, harder to sleep, and harder to find any motivation to take care of myself."

Although Jessi was surrounded by people every day, she felt deeply disconnected—from them, from herself, and from her own body. Naming her experience through the lens of the nervous system gave her something she hadn't had in a long time: compassion. Instead of blaming herself for the eating patterns she couldn't seem to stop, she began to understand them as adaptive responses from a nervous system doing its best to survive.

"It's like I'm trying to wake myself up," she said. "But it's not working." This insight didn't erase the exhaustion overnight or immediately change her behaviors, but it gave her a starting point. Jessi realized that what she needed most wasn't more willpower or another strict meal plan; it was support, softness, and gentle ways to invite herself back into connection.

For the vast majority of my clients, change doesn't happen overnight or even in a linear pattern. I often share with my clients a drawing inspired by a social media meme. On one side is a straight line labeled "What We Think Change Should Look Like." It's the fantasy path: one decision, endless follow-through, and no setbacks. Many of us expect this kind of trajectory. It feels logical: Decide to change, and then simply follow through.

Change isn't linear.
Setbacks are part of the path.

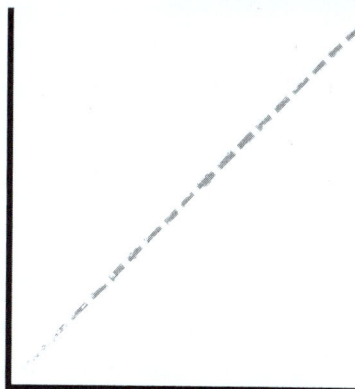

| **What We Think Change** | **What Change** |
| **Should Look Like** | **Actually Looks Like** |

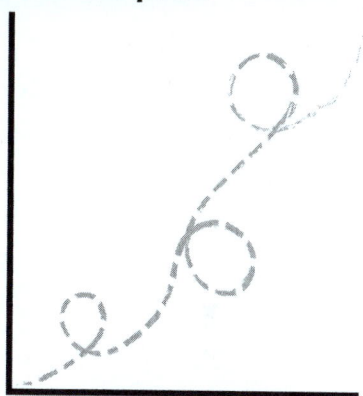

Change rarely follows a straight line. While we might expect progress to be a smooth climb, real transformation is full of loops, setbacks, and pauses. And that's not failure, that's being human.

On the other side of the drawing is a squiggly, looping line labeled "What Change Actually Looks Like." It twists and circles, sometimes doubling back or looping downward before moving forward again. This is what change looks like when it's happening inside a living, breathing body that moves through stress, joy, exhaustion, hunger, and connection—often in the same day. Food behaviors shift because states shift. When you're regulated, it might feel easy to nourish yourself intentionally. When you're dysregulated, your choices might default to survival strategies. That doesn't mean you're failing. It means your nervous system is doing what it's wired to do: protect you.

Changing How You Eat Is Different Than Changing Your Laundry Detergent

While progress isn't linear, every bit counts. The science of neuroplasticity tells us that the brain can make new connections and pathways when it learns and grows.

And trust me, there will be ups and downs. Unlike changing your laundry detergent, which only requires one decision whenever you need to buy more, changing how you engage with food is incredibly complex and involves thousands of decisions many times a day. Your food choices may shift based on the time of day, how hungry or full you feel, the rate of inflation, what foods you have available, whether you're tired, what season it is, how much movement you've done, your stress level, where you are in your menstrual cycle, and ten thousand other microscopic factors.

When we understand that our food choices are shaped by our nervous system states, we can begin to track something even deeper: our perspectives on food—what we value, prioritize, or feel drawn to—shift too.

In a regulated state, you might care about enjoying meals with friends, sustainability, or cooking from scratch. In sympathetic activation, you might prioritize accessibility, speed, or foods that regulate. In dorsal shutdown, you may just be trying to keep things simple, low effort, or safe. These shifts aren't flaws or inconsistencies; they're signals. Each state comes with its own set of needs, and your food values reflect what your body is asking for in that moment.

You don't have to eat the same way every day. Follow the rhythm of your nervous system.

How to Navigate Food

Survival Food Tool Kit

Ventral Regulation Food Tool Kit

When Things Are Tough

When You Have Capacity

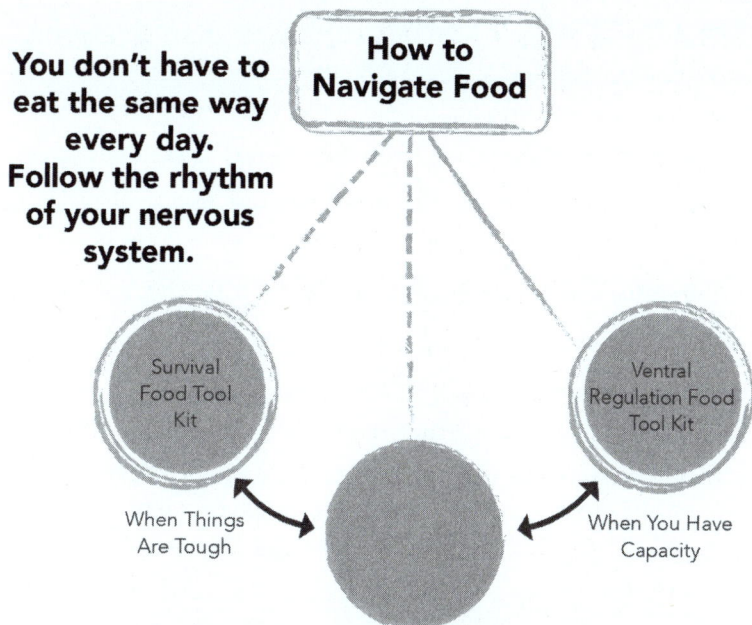

Your food needs change with your nervous system state. Instead of forcing one approach, build two tool kits. One for when you're regulated, and another for when you're just trying to get through the day.

Once you can start to name those shifting food perspectives, you can begin to build something incredibly helpful: a nutrition tool kit that's tailored to each state. Not a one-size fits-all approach, but a flexible, compassionate collection of options—foods, meal styles, preparation strategies—that support your body and nervous system *right where you are.*

Instead of trying to eat the "same way every day," this approach invites you to ask, "What does my nervous system value in this state? What matters to me when I'm here? What kind of food, or food experience, might support me right now?"

Let's start by naming those perspective shifts. Following is a list of food values that often show up across regulated and survival states. You may recognize some of them when you're feeling great and others when you're stressed, collapsed, or trying to get through the day. As you read through the list, notice that none of these values are morally "better" or "worse" than the others. For example, "accessible" isn't less valuable than "healthy"—it's just what matters more to you in a particular moment.

Going back to your What's Cooking in Your Nervous System diagram, choose words that describe your approach to food when you're in an activated state. Now choose three words that match your approach to food while in a "too low energy" dorsal shutdown state. In the next chapter, we'll fully flesh out our approach to food when we're regulated.

Accessible				
Available	Practical		**Some Possible**	
Easy	Simple	Efficient	**Approaches**	
Low effort	Storable	Comfort	**to Food**	
Fast	Affordable	Satisfying		
Convenient	Adaptable	Satiating		
Possible	Flexible	Normal	Self-expressive	Emotional connection
Reliable	Functional	Nourishing	From scratch	Natural
Safe	Minimal waste	Mindful	Creative	Minimally processed
Intuitive	Authentic	Farm-to-table	Artistic	Non-GMO
Traditional	International	Locally sourced	Inventive	Nutrient density
Family	Sustainable	Biodiversity	Balanced	Healthy
Community	Ethical	Organic	Variety	Budget-friendly

The story you tell yourself about food shifts with your nervous system state—because story follows state. This list helps you name the perspectives that may guide your choices in different moments, whether you're in ventral regulation or in a survival state. There's no right or wrong; just pick some approaches that reflect where you are.

Once you've chosen your three food perspectives for each nervous system state, take a few minutes to reflect on what you've discovered. Are there terms that show up across multiple states—things that remain important to you no matter how you're feeling? Are there values that seem to disappear entirely when you're in a survival state, such as cooking from scratch, eating healthy, or novelty?

Use Your Three Food Perspectives as a Compass

Once you've identified the food approaches that show up in each nervous system state, you can begin using them as a guide—rather than fighting against your current experience. For example, if your sympathetic activation-state values are "fast, filling, accessible," then expecting yourself to prepare a complex, home-cooked dinner isn't just unrealistic—it's likely to increase stress. Instead, choose meals that align with what your body is asking for in that state. A microwavable burrito, a smoothie with protein powder, or a handful of snacks you can assemble quickly may meet your needs more effectively than attempting the latest aspirational TikTok recipe.

Keeping your personal food approaches in mind, let's explore how to create a food tool kit you can lean on during survival states. There's no one "right" way to build this tool kit; everyone's needs and preferences are different. In fact, I've never had two clients design theirs the same way. What they *do* have in common is this: They plan ahead while in a regulated state, when their mind feels clearer and better resourced. Doing the mental work in advance can reduce decision fatigue and make it easier to care for yourself when you're overwhelmed, exhausted, or checked out.

How to Build a Workable Tool Kit for Survival States

As you read through the tool kit ideas below, consider which make sense for your life, your body, and your current season. You don't need to use every tool—just choose the ones that feel most helpful right now. And remember, you can build more than one tool kit for different situations or states.

Make a Flexible Meal Plan

When you're in a survival state—stressed, exhausted, or shut down—it can be incredibly hard to make decisions about food in the moment. That's why part of building your food tool kit is writing things down *before* you need them. Think of this as preparing a road map for the version of you who feels underwater. You're not creating a rigid plan—you're creating flexible, compassionate options for your future self to lean on. As you read through the following ideas, jot down the ones that feel most useful. Save them in your phone, stick them on your fridge, or keep them in a notes app labeled "Survival Food Tool Kit" so they're ready when you need them most.

- **Eating at a restaurant.** Make a list of a few restaurants where you feel comfortable and can get a satisfying meal without too much decision-making. This might be a favorite local spot, a chain where you know the menu by heart, or anywhere that feels low pressure. Eating out can offer relief from prep and cleanup and provide a small moment of connection or normalcy.

- **Getting takeout or delivery.** Save two to three go-to food delivery orders in your phone so you don't have to think about what to get when you're drained. Choose meals that feel grounding and supportive—things you know your body tolerates well and that don't leave you feeling worse after. Keep the names of restaurants or order links handy so they're just a few taps away.

- **Simple assembly meals using shortcuts like frozen rice, prechopped veggies, and cooked proteins.** These are meals you can pull together in five to ten minutes with minimal effort—just heat, combine, and eat. Keep a list of three to five easy combos that you like (for example: frozen rice, rotisserie chicken, salad greens, dressing). You can even write down where you usually buy the components to make restocking easier.

- **Backup meals from frozen or pantry items.** These are your emergency rations: the food you turn to when the fridge is empty and the idea of grocery shopping is overwhelming. Think shelf-stable soups, instant oats, canned beans, pasta, frozen burritos, or microwaveable bowls. Write out your top three to five backup meals so you don't have to think twice when you need them.

- **Snack-style meals if cooking feels too hard.** Snack meals are completely valid. When you don't have the capacity to cook, your goal is simply to get fed. Create a short list of mix-and-match options that work for you—things like boiled eggs, cheese sticks, crackers, fruit, hummus, or nut butter. You might even create a "snack plate template" with a protein, a carb, and a fruit or veggie.

Make a Grocery List That Includes Supportive, Low-Effort Options

Part of building a food tool kit is thinking ahead to what will actually feel doable when your energy is low. When you're in a survival state, even writing a grocery list or walking into a store can feel overwhelming, so let's take that decision-making off your plate now. Here are some key categories to include:

- **Single-serving items that are easy to eat.** These are grab-and-go foods that don't require prep, thought, or utensils—perfect for when you're too overwhelmed to cook. Some great options are individual yogurt cups, string cheese, apples or bananas, precut fruit, hummus and crackers, guacamole and tortilla chips, trail mix, granola bars, or shelf-stable protein shakes.

- **Assembly ingredients.** Stock up on foods that can be easily combined into a meal with little to no cooking. Think rotisserie chicken, bagged salad mixes, your favorite salad dressing, cooked lentils, hardboiled eggs, precooked rice or grains, and prewashed greens. Bonus if the components work across multiple meals.

- **Pre-made or heat-and-eat meals you like.** These are your "no energy" meals—things you can pop in the microwave or oven and have ready in minutes. Frozen burritos, grain bowls, soups, or prepared meals from your grocery store's deli section are all great options. Make sure you buy what you *actually like*; there's no point in stocking food that you don't like to eat.

- **Paper plates or cups.** Don't underestimate the power of reducing friction. If doing dishes is a barrier to eating, paper plates, cups, or even compostable utensils can be game-changers. It's not wasteful to care for yourself in a way that makes eating more accessible.

- **Other regularly needed household items.** Add essentials such as toilet paper, paper towels, soap, toothpaste, or anything else you might need. It's hard to think clearly about meals when you're also out of basic supplies. Keeping these stocked reduces one more layer of stress during hard times.

Whether you use Instacart, Amazon Fresh, or a local grocery store app, take a few minutes to build a "survival mode" grocery list. When things feel hard, you won't need to start from scratch—you'll just tap *order*.

Prepurchase: Stock Up Before the Hard Days Hit (If and When It's Possible)

One of the most supportive things you can do for yourself is to prepare for dysregulation while you're still in a regulated state. That said, prepurchasing depends on resources—not just time and energy but money too. If it's financially possible to buy a few extra items when you're grocery shopping, you can slowly build a buffer that your future self will be grateful for. It doesn't have to be expensive or purchased all at once. If you do have the ability to stock up ahead, here are some helpful items to keep in your tool kit:

- **Keep a few frozen meals in your freezer for backup.** Frozen meals are a low-effort safety net on days when cooking or planning feels like too much. Choose one or two you enjoy and keep them tucked away for a hard day. Even just one frozen burrito or pasta bowl in the freezer can be the difference between eating something or nothing.

- **Store shelf-stable basics in your pantry.** Little by little, add low-cost, long-lasting foods like canned beans, soups, peanut butter, rice, pasta, tuna, or instant oats. These pantry staples can become a full meal when fresh groceries run low, and they don't require refrigeration or fast use.

- **Try frozen veggies or steamable rice for fast, nutrient-dense options.** Frozen produce can be more affordable than fresh and lasts much longer. Steamable bags of rice, cauliflower, or mixed vegetables are perfect for quick meals when you're low on energy. Pair them with a canned or precooked protein such as canned tuna or frozen meatballs for something fast and nourishing.

- **Have emergency snacks in your bag, car, or desk for long days or unexpected delays.** Even a single granola bar tucked into your car's glove box or your backpack can make a difference on a tough day. If you're able, buy a few shelf-stable snacks when they're on sale—trail mix, protein bars, jerky, crackers, or dried fruit—and keep them in an accessible location.

If money is tight, your tool kit can still exist—just in different ways. You might focus on keeping the ingredients for one staple meal you love. It's okay to build slowly. In the meantime, I'd recommend downloading Leanne Brown's free cookbook, *Good and Cheap: Eat Well on $4/Day*. It's available on her website at: leannebrown.com/good-and-cheap-2/.

Reduce Decision Fatigue: Simplify Choices for Your Future Self

When you're in a survival state—whether overwhelmed, shut down, or simply out of bandwidth—decision-making can feel impossible. The mental load of figuring out *what to eat* becomes just one more thing your nervous system can't carry. That's why a key part of your food tool kit is doing that thinking *ahead of time* when you're in a more regulated state. By creating systems now, you make food more accessible and compassionate later. Here are some ways to reduce decision fatigue around meals:

- **Create a list of go-to meals and tape it inside a kitchen cabinet door.** Include three to five meals you can make with minimal effort and ingredients you usually have on hand. Think: scrambled eggs and toast, pasta with jarred sauce, quesadilla and fruit, or smoothie and granola. This visual reminder saves brainpower in the moment.

- **Rotate the same two to three breakfasts and lunches.** Pick a few go-to options you like and repeat them during the week. This works especially well for meals you eat alone. Save variety for when you have more energy or shared meals.

- **Use your favorite AI tool to generate recipe ideas based on what you have.** When you're low on energy and creativity, let technology do the work. Open your preferred AI assistant (such as ChatGPT, a recipe app, or Google Assistant), and type in a quick list of what's in your kitchen—for example, "I have canned black beans, rice, shredded cheese, and salsa." In seconds, you'll get recipe ideas you might not have thought of, like burrito bowls, stuffed peppers, or quesadillas. It's like having a meal-planning buddy who never gets tired.

Create Gentle Reminders and Set Alarms (Even If You Don't Turn Them on Yet)

When you're dysregulated, time can become hard to track—meals might get delayed, skipped, or forgotten entirely as stress or dorsal shutdown takes over. If that sounds familiar, it can be helpful to create a set of gentle, premade alarms on your phone to remind you to eat. You don't need to keep them on all the time, but when you're in survival mode, having them ready to activate with a single tap can be powerful. These reminders aren't meant to pressure or shame—they're soft cues to help you reconnect with your body's basic needs.

Here are a few supportive options to consider:

- Regular alarms for meals and snacks at times that match your usual routine
- A weekly reminder to restock essentials or place a grocery order
- Gentle daily check-ins like "Did I eat lunch today?" or "How's my energy?"

Even if you don't use them right away, setting up these reminders now means future you will have one less decision to make—and one more layer of support in place.

Involve Your Community: Make Connection Part of Your Care Plan

So often, when we're in a survival state, it feels like we have to do everything alone. Hyper-independence often shows up as a trauma response and we feel like it's safer not to rely on anyone. For many of us, there's also a cultural tension between doing it all ourselves and leaning on our community. Whether that shift to hyper-independence is rooted in trauma, generational expectations, or a cultural pressure to be self-sufficient, it's real and it's exhausting.

But community care is just as essential as self-care—and asking for support is a strength, not a weakness. Just because you can do it yourself doesn't mean you have to. Part of building your food tool kit is identifying ways others can support you when you don't have the capacity to manage food on your own.

Hyper-Independence	Trauma's Influence	Community Care
Do everything yourself, even when overwhelmed.	←	Ask for help with one small thing—such as a grocery pickup or check-in text.
Cook every meal from scratch, regardless of how drained you feel.	←	Trade meals with a friend or accept a dropped-off dinner.
Don't tell anyone you're struggling—keep it to yourself.	←	Let one trusted person know you're having a hard week.
Push through exhaustion without adjusting your expectations.	←	Outsource something—groceries, meal prep, childcare, cleaning
Hold the belief: "If I can do it, I should do it."	←	Adopt the mindset: "Just because I can doesn't mean I have to."
Avoid asking for help because it feels like weakness or burdening others.	←	See asking for help as a skill—and part of your wellness tool kit.

Hyper-independence often forms as a survival strategy. But over time, it can limit the support we need to truly heal. Practicing community care can be a powerful support to your nervous system.

It's also true that community isn't always simple or trigger free. Relationships can be messy. People may annoy you, misunderstand you, or bother you—but investing in community is a great way to grow your nervous system resilience. What would it look like to expand your "capacity circle" by including others in your care plan—not as a last resort, but as a sustainable practice?

This doesn't have to be complicated or dramatic, and it doesn't have to be all or nothing. Sometimes the smallest bit of help—a grocery pickup, a dropped-off meal, or even a check-in text—can make a big difference.

Here are a few ways to make community support more accessible:

- **Write a short message in your phone's notes that you can easily copy and paste when you need help.** That way, when you're too overwhelmed to explain, the words are already there. For example: *"Hey, things are a bit rough this week—would you be open to grabbing me a few grocery items or dropping off a meal?"*
  Having it saved removes the barrier of trying to find the right words when you're struggling.

- **Let someone you trust know what your fallback foods are and when they might check in.** You could say, "If I seem off or you haven't heard from me, it helps to ask if I've eaten. My go-to foods are frozen burritos, soup, and peanut butter toast." Giving someone that info ahead of time makes it easier for them to show up in a way that actually helps.

- **Trade support with a friend.** Set up a buddy system where you take turns helping each other through tough stretches—dropping off freezer meals, brainstorming low-effort dinners, or even just texting, "Have you eaten today?" Shared care builds accountability, reduces shame, and reminds you that you're not alone.

Community support isn't just a backup plan—it's part of the healing process. When others help you eat, they're also reminding you that you're worth feeding, even when you don't feel like it.

As you reach the end of this chapter, pause to look over what you've created. This tool kit isn't just a list of food hacks—it's a reflection of your deeper needs, shaped by your lived experiences, your nervous system states, and your wisdom about what helps you through hard times. When life gets hard (and it will), you now have something solid to return to, a system that says, "I know myself. I know what helps. I've thought about this already. I'm not starting from scratch."

CHAPTER 12

Building Your Ventral Regulation Nutrition Tool Kit

Transformation does not happen when
we do what we're told.
Transformation happens when we own
what we know to be true, and move
toward it.

—Abby Wambach, *Wolfpack*

Now that you've explored your experiences in survival states, it's time to turn toward something different: ventral regulation. Ventral regulation is the state of connection, presence, and true self. It's where you feel most like yourself—and where you have real choice.

In ventral regulation, you have the capacity to *choose* the approach to food that best supports you—not out of fear, urgency, or dorsal shutdown but out of true care. You can choose to nourish your body with colorful vegetables, quality proteins, and foods that promote long-term well-being. You can also choose to enjoy a sweet treat, a cozy meal, or a special occasion food without guilt or shame.

In ventral regulation, eating a salad and eating a cupcake can both come from the same grounded place; the difference isn't the food itself but the energy and intention behind the choice.

From ventral regulation, food becomes flexible, supportive, and connected to your real needs. You can tune in to what your body needs now and what it might need later and make choices that honor both. Ventral regulation isn't about eating "perfectly"; it's about having the freedom to nourish yourself in ways that feel good today and support your health into the future. It's about building a relationship with food that reflects trust, respect, and care for your body over time.

Now, pull out another piece of paper, and write the prompts as shown here:

What's Cooking in Your Nervous System?

Ventral Regulation

I know I'm in this state because	_____
Food is	_____
My chosen responses to food are	_____
Some ripple effects are	_____
Three words that describe my approach to food in this state are	_____

When you're in a state of ventral regulation, your approach to foods shifts from reactivity to choice. This activity helps you reflect on how foods feel when you're regulated, connected, and supported to your full capacity.

I know I'm in this state because . . .

When you're in a regulated state, you can usually feel the difference in both your body and your mind. Things slow down in a comfortable way. The world feels more manageable, even if it isn't perfect. You may notice a deeper connection to yourself and to others and a sense that you can meet challenges without becoming overwhelmed. This doesn't mean everything feels easy—it means you trust your capacity to respond.

You might notice:

- "The world is okay, and I can handle it."
- "I feel present and steady."
- "I can take a deep breath when something stressful happens."
- "I don't feel rushed or like I'm bracing for something bad."
- "I notice I'm more curious about things around me."

Food is . . .

In ventral regulation, your relationship with food often feels grounded, intentional, and flexible. Food doesn't carry the same urgency or emotional charge it might in survival states. Instead, food becomes part of how you care for yourself, supporting your energy, connection, and joy. Eating can feel satisfying, pleasurable, and responsive to your body's real needs. You might describe food as:

- "Food is nourishing and supportive."
- "Food is something I can enjoy without guilt."
- "Food is flexible—I can make different choices without stress."
- "Food is a way to care for my body and honor what it needs."
- "Food is a part of connection with people I love."

My chosen responses to food are . . .

When you're regulated, your responses to food feel more intentional, kind, and balanced. Instead of reacting automatically or rigidly, you can make food choices that match your values and needs in the moment. You might find yourself choosing both nutrient-dense foods and comfort foods with ease without falling into all-or-nothing thinking. In this state, you might notice your chosen responses are:

- "I choose meals that balance what my body needs now and later."
- "I include a variety of foods that nourish me and also bring me joy."
- "I pause and check in with my hunger or fullness before eating."
- "I let myself enjoy sweet treats without guilt when I want them."
- "I prepare meals that feel good and satisfy me."

Some ripple effects are . . .

The benefits of regulated eating extend beyond mealtimes. You might notice improvements physically, emotionally, or even in your relationships with others when you make food decisions from a place of connection and self-trust. The ripple effects often build gently over time, reinforcing your sense of well-being. Some ripple effects you might notice:

- "My energy throughout the day is steady instead of crashing."
- "I feel satisfied after eating instead of stuffed or deprived."
- "I spend less time obsessing over food or body image."
- "My digestion feels easier and more comfortable."
- "I'm more present during meals and less distracted."
- "I feel proud of how I'm caring for my body without perfectionism."

As you may remember, Jessi, a twenty-eight-year-old graduate student in social work, first explored her relationship with food when she was deep in dorsal shutdown energy. At the time, Jessi felt completely numb, moving through her days on autopilot, skipping meals without meaning to, and then eating at night in a disconnected haze. Food wasn't something she looked forward to; it was something she either forgot about or ate to try to feel something, anything, after long days that left her overwhelmed and depleted.

Over time, Jessi began to notice small, early signs that dorsal shutdown was starting to creep in. When she caught herself skipping meals during the day or rushing through conversations with other students, she would use the alarms she had preset on her phone to remind herself to eat. She also asked a friend to go grocery shopping with her, making it easier to stock up on simple, heat-and-eat meals. As Jessi learned to care for herself even while in a survival state, she found herself stuck there less and less.

After a few months, Jessi had experienced ventral regulation often enough that it felt like the right time to start building a Ventral Regulation Food Tool Kit. To begin, I asked her to work through the following prompts:

I know I'm in this state because . . .

- "The world is okay, and I can handle it."
- "I feel steady and don't have to rush through everything."
- "I can breathe deeper and feel more connected to myself."

Food is . . .

- "Food is nourishing and supportive."
- "Food is something I can actually enjoy."
- "Food is flexible—I can make choices without beating myself up."

My chosen responses to food are . . .

- "I choose foods that give me steady energy and actually taste good."
- "I include vegetables, but I also let myself have foods that feel comforting."
- "I listen to my hunger cues instead of ignoring them."

Some ripple effects are . . .

The benefits extended beyond eating itself.

- "I feel more even throughout the day—no more crashing and burning."
- "I don't obsess about food choices afterward."
- "I feel proud of how I'm treating my body."

Next, I asked Jessi to come up with three words that captured how she approaches food when she's regulated. She could choose from a list I gave her or come up with her own.

Accessible				
Available	Practical		**Some Possible**	
Easy	Simple	Efficient	**Approaches**	
Low effort	Storable	Comfort	**to Food**	
Fast	Affordable	Satisfying		
Convenient	Adaptable	Satiating		
Possible	Flexible	Normal	Self-expressive	Emotional connection
Reliable	Functional	Nourishing	From scratch	Natural
Safe	Minimal waste	Mindful	Creative	Minimally processed
Intuitive	Authentic	Farm-to-table	Artistic	Non-GMO
Traditional	International	Locally sourced	Inventive	Nutrient density
Family	Sustainable	Biodiversity	Balanced	Healthy
Community	Ethical	Organic	Variety	Budget-friendly

In the last chapter, you explored your food perspectives through the lens of survival. Now, from the connected energy of ventral regulation, take another look. What words resonate with you in this state? What becomes possible when you have the ability to choose and connect with your needs?

Jessi took a few minutes to think it over, then picked two words from my list—*healthy* and *practical*—and added one of her own: *fun*.

I asked her to tell me what that looked like and how it was different from her approach to food when in a survival state.

Jessi smiled as she shared the words she chose. *Fun* hadn't even been part of the picture before. When she was stuck in dorsal shutdown, food was either something she forgot about entirely or something she used just to get through the day. It wasn't something she enjoyed.

When we talked more about what *healthy* meant to her, Jessi explained that it meant caring for her future self. With a strong family history of diabetes, she had always been scared for her future health, but survival mode made it hard to act on that awareness. When she was regulated, it felt more natural to reach for foods that supported her health. She genuinely liked vegetables and nourishing meals; she simply lost track of them when she was overwhelmed.

Fun took on a specific and personal meaning too. For Jessi, it wasn't about expensive or elaborate experiences. Fun showed up in small things: picking up a specialty sauce from the grocery store to make everyday meals feel a little more exciting or checking out new, inexpensive restaurants with friends. Those little touches helped food feel less like another chore and more like something she could actually enjoy.

Practical aspects remained just as important. As a graduate student, it was rare for her to have the time or resources to cook elaborate meals or follow complicated nutrition plans. She valued having simple, realistic foods on hand—meals she could easily pull together, even on the busiest days, without slipping back into dorsal shutdown.

When she reflected on the difference between how she approached food in survival versus ventral regulation, the shift was clear. In survival, food was about getting by—eating whatever was quickest or easiest to numb the discomfort. In ventral regulation, food became about nourishment, ease, and a little bit of joy.

Stretch, Not Stress: Using Regulated Energy to Support Your Body

Because choice is possible in a regulated state, you have the space to pause, reflect, and try something new.

To guide this process, we'll borrow and modify a concept from polyvagal therapist Deb Dana, called the *Stress vs. Stretch Continuum*. It's a framework that helps you discern which actions feel like nourishing growth (*a stretch*) versus which feel overwhelming or dysregulating (*a stress*). A stretch feels slightly effortful, maybe a little new—but still accessible within a regulated energy state. A stress, on the other hand, pushes you too far, too fast, often triggering a survival state.

Think of it like this:

Stretch = a gentle challenge, a fun experiment, a supportive step forward

Stress = a demand that exceeds your current capacity, leading to avoidance or disconnection

This idea—that there's a sweet spot between not enough challenge and too much—isn't new. In fact, it echoes the Yerkes-Dodson Law, first proposed by psychologists Robert Yerkes and John Dodson in 1908. They discovered that a little bit of stress can help us focus and perform better—but only up to a point. When the stress level gets too high, it starts to work against us. This idea is often shown as an upside-down U: too little stress, and we feel unmotivated; too much, and we feel overwhelmed. But in the middle, there's a sweet spot where we feel alert, capable, and able to take action.

Yerkes-Dodson Law
Not all stress is bad, some can help us focus and take action. Finding the right amount is crucial.

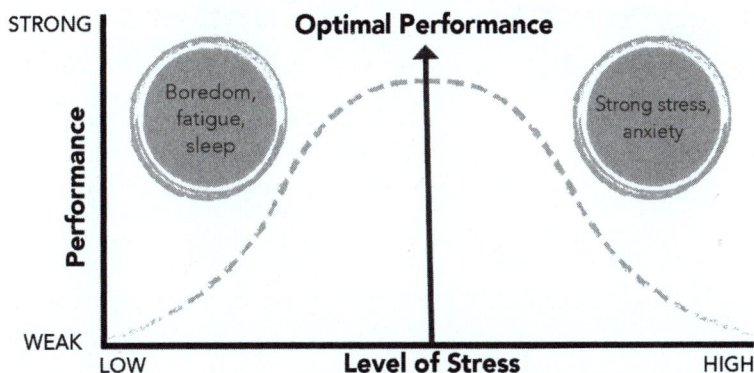

Remember to choose experiments with food that are a stretch, not a stress to your nervous system. What feels like a stretch one day may feel overwhelming and stressful the next and that's okay. Let your nervous system state be your guide.

When viewed through a polyvagal lens, this sweet spot often reflects a blend of regulated and activated energy—just enough ventral/sympathetic blend to spark motivation, playfulness, and experimentation, but not too much to send us into a true survival state. Think of this blend as the difference between curiosity and urgency.

Here's how you can use this framework to support your body. First, pull out the What's Cooking in Your Nervous System paper and look at the section on ventral regulation. If you haven't already, fill out three words that best reflect the approach you'd like to have to food when regulated. Next, look back at the tools from Part II of the book and consider whether any of the ideas in those chapters would fit within your framework as a stretch, not a stress.

Need a refresher?

From Chapter 5:

- Try balancing your meals with a mix of protein, fats, and carbs that sustain your energy.
- Begin to include more protein in your meals, especially at breakfast or lunch.
- Add foods rich in omega-3s, such as salmon, walnuts, or chia seeds.
- Include more vitamin D, iron, zinc, magnesium, or B vitamins—either through food or supplementation, if needed.
- Experiment with fueling your body for energy—not just survival.

From Chapter 7:

- Reconnect with others—have a meal with someone supportive or cuddle with your pet.
- Spend time in nature—even a short walk, open window, or potted plant can offer grounding.
- Try breathwork or a moment of mindfulness.
- Prioritize restorative sleep by winding down with a calming snack, herbal tea, or screen-free time.
- Support relaxation by taking a warm bath or shower and consider sauna therapy if accessible to you.
- Schedule an often-overlooked form of care, such as going to the dentist or a physical with your primary care provider.
- Explore gentle movement, such as stretching, walking, or dancing to music, as a way to reconnect to your body.
- Add more anti-inflammatory foods to meals, such as turmeric, berries, leafy greens, or olive oil.

From Chapter 9:

- Practice digestive hygiene: Slow down, chew well, and eat without multitasking.
- Add fiber-rich foods such as oats, lentils, berries, or flaxseeds to meals.
- Explore polyphenol-rich foods such as pomegranate, green tea, or dark chocolate.
- Include probiotic foods such as yogurt, kefir, kimchi, or pickles.
- Diversify your diet: Try one new fruit, vegetable, or whole food this week to support your gut microbiome.

Choosing the right experiment (or experiments) isn't just about picking the individual actions that feel like a stretch rather than a stress. It's also about how many experiments you choose to try at once. Even if each action on its own feels completely manageable, trying to do *everything* on the list at once can overwhelm your system and nudge you right back into a survival state.

Only you can sense what's supportive right now. No influencer or expert can feel your internal state. Choose experiments that keep you anchored in ventral.

How I Want You to Choose Your Nutrition Experiments

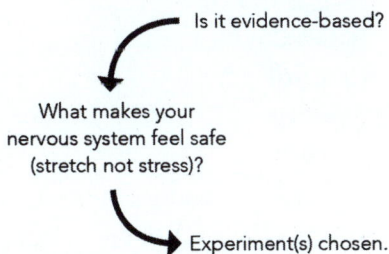

Is it evidence-based?

What makes your nervous system feel safe (stretch not stress)?

Experiment(s) chosen.

Choosing the right nutrition experiment starts with noticing and naming your own nervous system state. And no one, including the wellness influencers on social media or even your best friend, can determine that for you. What feels like a "stretch, not a stress" will be unique to you, and that's exactly the point.

It's easy to slip from curiosity into urgency without even realizing it—especially when you're feeling excited or hopeful about change.

Instead of treating these ideas like a to-do list you must check off, think of them as a menu.

Your goal isn't to choose everything. Your goal is to choose one or two stretches that feel nourishing, sustainable, and kind to your current capacity. You can always come back and add more experiments later—once the first few become part of your natural daily flow.

When you've chosen one or two stretch goals—like eating more vegetables, walking in nature, or sitting down to eat—I want you to picture them on a battery that charges and drains depending on your nervous system capacity. While we aim to spend more time in ventral regulation, we can't expect our battery to stay full all the time. That's why it helps to map your stretch goals across a spectrum, from the easiest, most energy-conserving version to the most demanding. On days when your battery is running low, you can stick to the gentlest, most doable version. On days when you feel more charged up and regulated, you might choose to push a little further. Here's what that could look like using the example of eating more vegetables:

Stretch or Stress?

What works for your nervous system today?

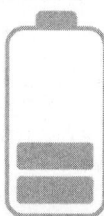

Order pizza and a salad.	Toss frozen vegetables into meals you're already making.	Lightly prep raw veggies for snacks or simple sides.	Cook a basic vegetable dish alongside your main meal.	Plan and cook a full, vegetable-heavy recipe from scratch.

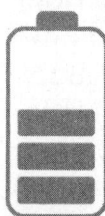

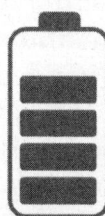

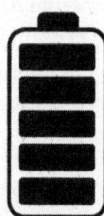

Stretch looks different depending on your battery level. This visual maps one goal—eating more vegetables—across different effort levels. On low-energy days, the easiest version still counts as progress. On more resourced days, you might choose to stretch a bit further.

Stretch to Stress Spectrum: Adding Vegetables

- **Easiest Stretch.** Add a veggie side to something you're already ordering or eating.
- **Easy Stretch.** Eat prewashed, precut vegetables straight from the package.
- **Moderate Stretch.** Toss raw or frozen vegetables into meals you're already making.
- **Moderate to Challenging Stretch.** Prep raw veggies for snacks or simple sides.
- **Challenging Stretch.** Cook a basic vegetable dish alongside your main meal.
- **Most Difficult/Stress.** Plan and cook a full, vegetable-heavy recipe from scratch.

Just as with adding vegetables, you can apply the stretch-to-stress spectrum to nearly any supportive habit. The goal isn't to hit the "most difficult" version every time; it's to find an entry point that feels accessible based on your current nervous system state. On regulated days, you might feel up for a bigger challenge. On survival days, the tiniest version still counts. Let's look at how this same spectrum might apply to the goal of walking in nature.

Stretch to Stress Spectrum: Walking in Nature

- **Easiest Stretch.** Step outside for two minutes and notice the sky, a tree, or a patch of grass.
- **Easy Stretch.** Take a short walk around the block or your building.
- **Moderate Stretch.** Walk for ten to fifteen minutes in a familiar outdoor space like a nearby park.
- **Moderate to Challenging Stretch.** Drive to a green space or trail and go for a longer, more intentional walk.

- **Challenging Stretch.** Plan a nature outing with a friend or family member that involves more time and energy.
- **Most Difficult Stress.** Commit to a structured hike or outdoor exercise class that requires gear, travel, or coordination.

You can build your own version of this model for any stretch goal. Grab a piece of paper and choose one experiment—or a few—that you'd like to try. Then, map out what that experiment looks like across your spectrum of nervous system capacity. Start with the easiest possible version you could do on a hard day and work your way up to what it might look like when you're feeling fully regulated and resourced. This exercise helps you build flexibility and self-compassion into your goals—so you can keep moving forward without burning out.

Experiment I'd Like to Focus on Now . . .

Easiest: _____

Easy: _____

Moderate: _____

Moderate to challenging: _____

Challenging: _____

Most difficult stretch: _____

Use this exercise to map your stretch goal across a spectrum—from the gentlest, least-effort version you can attempt on a hard day to the most ambitious one you'd try when you're feeling fully regulated and resourced.

What If You Don't Feel Regulated Yet?

For many people—especially those who have spent a long time living in survival states—ventral regulation isn't a familiar feeling.

You may not even remember a time when you felt grounded and safe.

If you don't feel regulated enough right now to build a food tool kit, that's completely normal. Your goal in this moment isn't to eat more vegetables or add more protein. Your goal is to find moments of ventral regulation—even tiny ones—in whatever ways feel most possible for you.

If imagining food from a place of safety and connection feels hard, you're not alone. For many people who have navigated food from sympathetic activation, dorsal shutdown, or survival for years, experiencing food through ventral regulation can feel unfamiliar or even out of reach. That's okay. You don't have to feel fully regulated to begin imagining what it might be like. Even the act of wondering—*What could food feel like if it felt safe?*—is a meaningful step toward change.

To understand why food can feel so complicated, it helps to consider a concept that therapist and educator Linda Thai calls *hashtags*.

In this context, hashtags refer to the way our nervous system unconsciously creates associations around certain experiences. For example, someone who survived a house fire might not only react to the fire itself but also to things like #smokyair, #burntsmell, #flickeringlight, or #midnightsilence—small sensory cues that became wired together with fear and loss.

In the same way, food can carry its own hashtags of distress.

Someone who grew up in a household where eating was monitored or criticized might now associate food with #shame, #weighins, #familydinners, or #cleanplateclub. Even years later, sitting down to a meal might trigger a protective survival response—not because the food itself is dangerous, but because it was once paired with feelings of being judged, unsafe, or not enough.

Finding Your Food Glimmers

Polyvagal therapist Deb Dana introduced the idea of *glimmers*—those small, often subtle cues that remind your nervous system you're safe, connected, and okay. Though our systems are wired to scan for #danger, we can teach them to notice glimmers of safety.

In this next exercise, we'll start identifying your food glimmers: the people, settings, textures, and small rituals that remind you that nourishment can feel possible.

Think about a satisfying meal.

Not just tasty but satisfying on every level—the right temperature, the right texture, the right feeling. You feel emotionally steady. Physically, you're comfortably full—not hungry again in thirty minutes but not so stuffed you feel bloated or sluggish.

If it's been a while since you had a meal like that, no problem. You can imagine it or think about what that experience might look like.

Once you have a meal in mind, start describing it:

Who was with you?

I'm guessing that your most recent satisfying meal probably wasn't with someone who annoys you. But who was there? Was it a good friend? A partner? Your family?

At your most satisfying meals, who's nearby?

- A good friend?
- A supportive partner?
- A pet quietly resting at your feet?
- Maybe you're happiest eating solo, savoring your own company.

Where were you?

Where you eat can quietly shape how safe and satisfied you feel.

Were you:

- At the kitchen table?
- Curled up on the couch?
- In the car between errands?
- Outside having a picnic?
- Maybe even eating in bed, if that feels most comforting.

What does your place setting look like?

Think about what you're eating from:

- A neatly arranged plate?
- A cozy bowl you can hold?
- Your hands, reaching for finger foods?

What tastes, textures, or temperatures do you like?

Sensory details can make a huge difference. Consider:

- Do you crave warm, cozy meals or refreshing, cold foods?
- Do you prefer soft, smooth textures or crunchy, layered ones?
- Do bold flavors excite you, or do gentle, familiar tastes feel best?

As you finish this glimmers exercise, take a moment to notice what elements stood out to you. What sensory cues, textures, or settings consistently help you feel more grounded, more comfortable, more yourself? These are your food glimmers—the small, personal details that signal safety and presence.

How could you include any of these glimmers more often in your meals, even in small ways? Would a certain utensil, a favorite spice, or music playing while you cook help bring a bit more ventral regulation into your routine? You might even consider weaving some of these elements into your survival-state food plans. A snack that's easy to eat *and* reminds you of comfort. A familiar dish served in a cozy spot. A moment of quiet before your first bite. Your food glimmers don't need to be saved for either your best or worst days; you can use them regularly to help point your nervous system to safety.

My best glimmer? Tacos. On a near weekly basis I make tacos from scratch. I can't say that this is the most authentic taco recipe. After all, I learned it from my mom in 1980s rural Iowa. But there is just something about making tacos that feels super regulating. It's half about how the tacos actually taste (delicious, naturally) and half about how I have to slow down to get the timing right in case I burn the taco shells while cutting up tomatoes. If you're not sure of your own food glimmers, I'd be really happy for you to try mine.

Probably Inauthentic
but Definitely Yummy Tacos

1 glug olive oil

½ onion, chopped

2 pounds ground beef

1 packet taco seasoning
OR the following:

> 1 tablespoon chili powder
>
> 1 teaspoon garlic powder
>
> 1 teaspoon onion powder
>
> ½ teaspoon oregano
>
> ¼ teaspoon cumin
>
> Salt and pepper to taste

1 can seasoned refried beans

2 tablespoons water

Taco shells and toppings to taste (salsa, guacamole, tomatoes, sour cream, black olives, lettuce)

DIRECTIONS:

1. Heat a sauté pan over medium heat, then put in a glug of olive oil.

2. Add onions and cook until soft, then add beef. If you have a fancy-pants ground meat tenderizer/mallet, use that to break apart the meat. Otherwise, make do with whatever tools you have.

3. Cook ground beef until brown. If your beef has a lot of fat in it, you can drain it or be daring and do what I do: put a paper towel right into the pan. (Use caution if you have a gas stove—don't want to catch that paper towel on fire!). Add the taco seasoning packet, the can of refried beans, and the water. Yes, this will be messy. That's part of the appeal; the stirring is relaxing.

4. Stir to incorporate and let heat through for a couple minutes.

5. In the meantime, put some taco shells in the oven as per package directions, and get ready to fill.

6. Fill your taco shells, add toppings as your heart guides, and enjoy!

Now You Have the Tools

You've covered a lot of ground throughout these pages. You've explored how survival states shape your relationship with food, how dorsal shutdown and sympathetic activation can pull you away from nourishment, and how ventral regulation can open the door to real choice, flexibility, and connection. You've seen how small shifts— such as building a Survival Nutrition Tool Kit, identifying your food glimmers, and choosing one stretch at a time—can create real, sustainable change.

You've learned that food isn't just fuel—or something to control with discipline. It's a way your nervous system communicates. It's a tool for building resilience. And it's one of the ways you can care for yourself, especially when life feels like too much. This work hasn't been about chasing the perfect diet or sticking to a rigid plan. It's been about learning to hear your body more clearly, respond with more kindness, and create a relationship with food that supports you instead of making you feel ashamed.

There is no one "perfect" path forward from here. There is only practice, curiosity, and compassion. Some days will feel easy. Some will feel messy. What matters is not whether you get it right every time, but that you come back to yourself with kindness. Every small moment of care you offer yourself matters more than you realize.

You are not broken. You are not behind. You are already on your way home to yourself. Every meal—whether it's a colorful salad, a comforting taco, or a warm mug of tea—is another opportunity to choose nourishment, foster connection, and trust in your own process.

Special Thanks

This book would not have been possible without the extraordinary community that surrounds me—colleagues, collaborators, and co-conspirators in the work of trauma-informed, nervous system–centered nutrition care.

To my brilliant business partners, Alyson Roux and Liz Abel, thank you for your unwavering faith in the work we do together, your thoughtful insights, and your deep commitment to transforming how nutrition is practiced and taught. I'm so grateful for your vision and the incredible community we've built together—a space grounded in integrity, collaboration, and care.

To my trusted colleagues—Nirvana Abdul-Gabal, Ashley Comparin, Leslie Castro-Woodhouse, Emily Cerda, Mary Virginia Coffman, Ariel Curry, Melanee Dahl, Rea Frey, Leah Haggard, Josie Kharitonenkov, Stephanie Lanham, Justein Mathias, Aaron Mlnarik, Tessa O'Toole, Amber Pawula-Marcin, Janine Rodrigues, Robin Ross, Cyndi Salemy, Amy Smith, Stephanie Thompson, Lauren Teeter, and Tina Zorger—thank you for the many ways you've influenced my thinking, supported my writing, and stood beside me as this vision became real.

A special call out to Jessica Thiefels, who transforms my wordy prose into concise images—couldn't have managed without you!

To my clients, thank you for sharing your stories and allowing me to hold space.

Thank you, especially, to Marilyn Allen and Christine Belleris, who believed in this idea from the very beginning—even when it was still rough around the edges. Your early support made all the difference.

And finally, to W and B, we're having tacos tonight.

Endnotes

Introduction

1. Fagan, J., Galea, S., Ahern, J., Bonner, S., & Vlahov, D. (2003). Relationship of self-reported asthma severity and urgent health care utilization to psychological sequelae of the September 11, 2001 terrorist attacks on the World Trade Center among New York City area residents. *Psychosomatic Medicine, 65*(6), 993–996. https://doi.org/10.1097/01 .PSY.0000097334.48556.5F

Chapter 1

1. Syed, K., & Iswara, K. (2023). Low-FODMAP diet. In *StatPearls*. StatPearls Publishing.

2. Altobelli, E., Del Negro, V., Angeletti, P. M., & Latella, G. (2017). Low-FODMAP diet improves irritable bowel syndrome symptoms: A meta-analysis. *Nutrients, 9*(9), 940. https://doi.org/ 10.3390/nu9090940

3. Van der Kolk, B. A. (2014). The body keeps the score: *Brain, mind, and body in the healing of trauma.* (p. 36). Viking.

4. Schafte, K., & Bruna, S. (2023). The influence of intergenerational trauma on epigenetics and obesity in Indigenous populations—a scoping review. *Epigenetics, 18*(1), 2260218. https://doi.org/10.1080/15592294.2023.2260218

5. Porges, S. W. (2022). Polyvagal theory: A science of safety. *Frontiers in Integrative Neuroscience, 16*, 871227. https://doi.org/10.3389/fnint.2022
    .871227

6. Prescott, S. L., & Liberles, S. D. (2022). Internal senses of the vagus nerve. *Neuron, 110*(4), 579–599. https://doi.org/10.1016/j.neuron.2021.12.020

7. Dana, D. (2023). *Polyvagal practices: anchoring the self in safety.* W. W. Norton & Company.

8. Maslow, A. H. (1943). A theory of human motivation. *Psychological Review, 50*(4), 370–396.

9. Van der Kolk, B. A. (2014). *The body keeps the score: Brain, mind, and body in the healing of trauma.* (p. 36). Viking.

10. Šimić, G., Tkalčić, M., Vukić, V., Mulc, D., Španić, E., Šagud, M., Olucha-Bordonau, F. E., Vukšić, M., & Hof, P. (2021). Understanding emotions: Origins and roles of the amygdala. *Biomolecules, 11*(6), 823. https://doi.org/10.3390/biom11060823

11. Porges, S. W. (2009). The polyvagal theory: New insights into adaptive reactions of the autonomic nervous system. *Cleveland Clinic Journal of Medicine, 76* Suppl 2(Suppl 2), S86–S90. https://doi.org/10.3949/ccjm.76.s2.17

12. Gordon, J. S. (2021). *Transforming trauma: The path to hope and healing.* HarperOne.

13. Lei, A. A., Phang, V. W. X., Lee, Y. Z., Kow, A. S. F., Tham, C. L., Ho, Y. C., & Lee, M. T. (2025). Chronic stress-associated depressive disorders: The impact of HPA axis dysregulation and neuroinflammation on the hippocampus—a mini review. *International Journal of Molecular Sciences, 26*(7), 2940. https://doi.org/10.3390/ijms26072940

14. Porges, S. W. (2022). Polyvagal theory: A science of safety. *Frontiers in Integrative Neuroscience, 16*, 871227. https://doi.org/10.3389/fnint.2022.871227

Chapter 2

1. Claes, S. J. (2004). Corticotropin-releasing hormone (CRH) in psychiatry: From stress to psychopathology. *Annals of Medicine, 36*(1), 50–61. https://doi.org/10.1080/07853890310017044

2. Sominsky, L., & Spencer, S. J. (2014). Eating behavior and stress: A pathway to obesity. *Frontiers in Psychology, 5*, 434. https://doi.org/10.3389/fpsyg.2014.00434

3. Sominsky, L., & Spencer, S. J. (2014). Eating behavior and stress: A pathway to obesity. *Frontiers in Psychology, 5*, 434. https://doi.org/10.3389/fpsyg.2014.00434

4. Sominsky, L., & Spencer, S. J. (2014). Eating behavior and stress: A pathway to obesity. *Frontiers in Psychology, 5,* 434. https://doi.org/10.3389/fpsyg.2014.00434

5. Lytvynenko, O., & König, L. M. (2024). Investigation of Ukrainian refugees' eating behavior, food intake, and psychological distress: Study protocol and baseline data. *Applied*

Psychology. Health and Well-Being, 16(3), 923–943. https://doi
.org/10.1111/aphw.12477

6. Raspopow, K., Abizaid, A., Matheson, K., & Anisman, H.
    (2010). Psychosocial stressor effects on cortisol and ghrelin in
    emotional and non-emotional eaters: influence of anger and
    shame. *Hormones and behavior, 58*(4), 677–684. https://doi.
    org/10.1016/j.yhbeh.2010.06.003

7. Dana, D. A. (2021). *Anchored: How to befriend your nervous
    system using polyvagal theory.* Sounds True.

Chapter 3

1. Moieni, M., Irwin, M. R., Jevtic, I., Breen, E. C., Cho, H. J.,
    Arevalo, J. M., Ma, J., Cole, S. W., & Eisenberger, N. I. (2015).
    Trait sensitivity to social disconnection enhances pro-
    inflammatory responses to a randomized controlled trial of
    endotoxin. *Psychoneuroendocrinology, 62*, 336–342. https://doi
    .org/10.1016/j.psyneuen.2015.08.020

2. Flaherty, S. C., & Sadler, L. S. (2011). A review of attachment
    theory in the context of adolescent parenting. *Journal of Pedi-
    atric Health Care, 25*(2), 114–121. https://doi.org/10.1016/j
    .pedhc.2010.02.005

3. Flaherty, S. C., & Sadler, L. S. (2011). A review of attachment
    theory in the context of adolescent parenting. *Journal of Pedi-
    atric Health Care, 25*(2), 114–121. https://doi.org/10.1016/j
    .pedhc.2010.02.005

4. Allen, J. (2013). *Mentalizing in the development and treatment
    of attachment trauma.* Karnac Books.

5. Brewerton, T. D. (2018). An overview of trauma-informed care and practice for eating disorders. *Journal of Aggression, Maltreatment & Trauma, 28*(4), 445–462. https://doi.org/10.1080/10926771.2018.1532940

6. Hazzard, V. M., Bauer, K. W., Mukherjee, B., Miller, A. L., & Sonneville, K. R. (2019). Associations between childhood maltreatment latent classes and eating disorder symptoms in a nationally representative sample of young adults in the United States. *Child Abuse & Neglect, 98,* 104171. https://doi.org/10.1016/j.chiabu.2019.104171

Chapter 4

1. Wang, L. J., Li, S. C., Li, S. W., Kuo, H. C., Lee, S. Y., Huang, L. H., Chin, C. Y., & Yang, C. Y. (2022). Gut microbiota and plasma cytokine levels in patients with attention-deficit/hyperactivity disorder. *Translational Psychiatry, 12*(1), 76. https://doi.org/10.1038/s41398-022-01844-x

2. Fasano, A., & Catassi, C. (2001). Current approaches to diagnosis and treatment of celiac disease: An evolving spectrum. *Gastroenterology, 120*(3), 636–651. https://doi.org/10.1053/gast.2001.22123

3. Volta, U., Bardella, M. T., Calabrò, A., Troncone, R., Corazza, G. R., & Study Group for Non-Celiac Gluten Sensitivity (2014). An Italian prospective multicenter survey on patients suspected of having non-celiac gluten sensitivity. *BMC Medicine, 12*, 85. https://doi.org/10.1186/1741-7015-12-85

4. Sanz Y. (2010). Effects of a gluten-free diet on gut microbiota and immune function in healthy adult humans. *Gut Microbes, 1*(3), 135–137. https://doi.org/10.4161/gmic.1.3.11868

Chapter 5

1. Ellis, P. (2020, August 20). James Blunt ate nothing but meat to prove how manly he was. Then he got scurvy. *Men's Health.* https://www.menshealth.com/entertainment/a33656947/james -blunt-carnivore-diet-scurvy/

2. Passarelli, S., Free, C., Shepon, A., Beal, T., Batis, C., & Golden, C. (2024). Global estimation of dietary micronutrient inadequacies: A modelling analysis. *The Lancet Global Health, 12*(10). https://doi.org/10.1016/S2214-109X(24)00276-6

3. Reider, C. A., Chung, R. Y., Devarshi, P. P., Grant, R. W., & Hazels Mitmesser, S. (2020). Inadequacy of immune health nutrients: Intakes in US adults, the 2005–2016 NHANES. *Nutrients, 12*(6), 1735. https://doi.org/10.3390/nu12061735

4. Yin, J., Gu, M., Zhou, Y., Wang, Y., Zhang, M., Yang, Y., Cai, Y., He, S., & Peng, D. (2025). Association of 24-h energy intake behavior with depressive symptoms: Findings from the National Health and Nutrition Examination Survey. *Depression and Anxiety, 2025,* 5544651. https://doi.org/10.1155/da/5544651

5. Silva, D., Mendes, F. C., Stanzani, V., Moreira, R., Pinto, M., Beltrão, M., Sokhatska, O., Severo, M., Padrão, P., Garcia-Larsen, V., Delgado, L., Moreira, A., & Moreira, P. (2025). The acute effects of a fast-food meal versus a Mediterranean food meal on the autonomic nervous system, lung function, and airway inflammation: A randomized crossover trial. *Nutrients, 17*(4), 614. https://doi.org/10.3390/nu17040614

6. Pachter, D., Kaplan, A., Tsaban, G., Zelicha, H., Meir, A. Y., Rinott, E., Levakov, G., Salti, M., Yovell, Y., Huhn, S., Beyer, F.,

Witte, V., Kovacs, P., von Bergen, M., Ceglarek, U., Blüher, M., Stumvoll, M., Hu, F. B., Stampfer, M. J., Friedman, A., … Shai, I. (2024). Glycemic control contributes to the neuroprotective effects of Mediterranean and green-Mediterranean diets on brain age: the DIRECT PLUS brain-magnetic resonance imaging randomized controlled trial. *The American Journal of Clinical Nutrition, 120*(5), 1029–1036. https://doi.org/10.1016/j .ajcnut.2024.09.013.

7. Zhang, H., Wang, Z., Wang, G., Song, X., Qian, Y., Liao, Z., Sui, L., Ai, L., & Xia, Y. (2023). Understanding the connection between gut homeostasis and psychological stress. *The Journal of Nutrition, 153*(4), 924–939. https://doi.org/10.1016/j.tjnut .2023.01.026

8. Dyall, S. C., Malau, I. A., & Su, K. P. (2025). Omega-3 polyunsaturated fatty acids in depression: Insights from recent clinical trials. *Current Opinion in Clinical Nutrition and Metabolic Care, 28*(2), 66–74. https://doi.org/10.1097/ MCO.0000000000001077

9. Sullivan, J. P., & Jones, M. K. (2024). The multifaceted impact of bioactive lipids on gut health and disease. *International Journal of Molecular Sciences, 25*(24), 13638. https://doi.org/10 .3390/ijms252413638

10. Lamon-Fava, S. (2025). Associations between omega-3 fatty acid–derived lipid mediators and markers of inflammation in older subjects with low-grade chronic inflammation. *Prosta-Glandins & Other Lipid Mediators, 176*, 106948. https://doi.org /10.1016/j.prostaglandins.2025.106948

11. Sproten, R., Nohr, D., & Guseva, D. (2024). Nutritional strategies modulating the gut microbiome as a preventative and therapeutic approach in normal and pathological age-related cognitive decline: A systematic review of preclinical and clinical findings. *Nutritional Neuroscience, 27*(9), 1042–1057. https://doi.org/10.1080/1028415X.2023.2296727

12. Sproten, R., Nohr, D., & Guseva, D. (2024). Nutritional strategies modulating the gut microbiome as a preventative and therapeutic approach in normal and pathological age-related cognitive decline: A systematic review of preclinical and clinical findings. *Nutritional Neuroscience, 27*(9), 1042–1057. https://doi.org/10.1080/1028415X.2023.2296727

13. Rubio, C., López-Landa, A., Romo-Parra, H., & Rubio-Osornio, M. (2025). Impact of the ketogenic diet on neurological diseases: A review. *Life (Basel, Switzerland), 15*(1), 71. https://doi.org/10.3390/life15010071

14. Medoro, A., Buonsenso, A., Centorbi, M., Calcagno, G., Scapagnini, G., Fiorilli, G., & Davinelli, S. (2024). Omega-3 index as a sport biomarker: Implications for cardiovascular health, injury prevention, and athletic performance. *Journal of functional morphology and kinesiology, 9*(2), 91. https://doi.org/10.3390/jfmk9020091

15. Bhardwaj, R. L., Parashar, A., Parewa, H. P., & Vyas, L. (2024). An alarming decline in the nutritional quality of foods: The biggest challenge for future generations' health. *Foods (Basel, Switzerland), 13*(6), 877. https://doi.org/10.3390/foods13060877

16. Storz, M. A., & Ronco, A. L. (2022). Nutrient intake in low-carbohydrate diets in comparison to the 2020-2025 Dietary Guidelines for Americans: A cross-sectional study. *The British Journal of Nutrition, 129*(6), 1–14. Advance online publication. https://doi.org/10.1017/S0007114522001908

17. Vici, G., Belli, L., Biondi, M., & Polzonetti, V. (2016). Gluten free diet and nutrient deficiencies: A review. *Clinical Nutrition (Edinburgh, Scotland), 35*(6), 1236–1241. https://doi.org/10.1016/j.clnu.2016.05.002

18. Mohan, M., Okeoma, C. M., & Sestak, K. (2020). Dietary gluten and neurodegeneration: A case for preclinical studies. *International Journal of Molecular Sciences, 21*(15), 5407. https://doi.org/10.3390/ijms21155407

19. Liu, L., Liu, S., Wang, C., Guan, W., Zhang, Y., Hu, W., Zhang, L., He, Y., Lu, J., Li, T., Liu, X., Xuan, Y., & Wang, P. (2019). Folate supplementation for methotrexate therapy in patients with rheumatoid arthritis: A systematic review. *Journal of Clinical Rheumatology: Practical Reports on Rheumatic & Musculoskeletal Diseases, 25*(5), 197–202. https://doi.org/10.1097/RHU.0000000000000810

20. Kaur, J., Khare, S., Sizar, O., et al. Vitamin D deficiency. [Updated 2025 Feb 15]. In: StatPearls [Internet]. Treasure Island (FL): StatPearls Publishing. Available from: https://www.ncbi.nlm.nih.gov/books/NBK532266/

21. Mordarski, B. (2023). *Nutrition-focused physical exam pocket guide* (3rd ed.). Academy of Nutrition and Dietetics.

22. National Institutes of Health, Office of Dietary Supplements. (2022, November 8). Vitamin D: Fact sheet for health

professionals. https://ods.od.nih.gov/factsheets/VitaminD
-HealthProfessional/

23. American Academy of Dermatology. (n.d.). Vitamin D: Position
statement. https://www.aad.org/media/stats-vitamin-d

24. Baswan, S. M., Klosner, A. E., Weir, C., Salter-Venzon, D.,
Gellenbeck, K. W., Leverett, J., & Krutmann, J. (2021). Role of
ingestible carotenoids in skin protection: A review of clinical
evidence. *Photodermatology, Photoimmunology & Photomedi-
cine, 37*(6), 490–504. https://doi.org/10.1111/phpp.12690

25. Cashman, K. D. (2022). Global differences in vitamin D status
and dietary intake: A review of the data. *Endocrine Connections, 11*(1), e210282. https://doi.org/10.1530/EC-21-0282

26. Cardwell, G., Bornman, J. F., James, A. P., & Black, L. J. (2018).
A review of mushrooms as a potential source of dietary vitamin
D. *Nutrients, 10*(10), 1498. https://doi.org/10.3390/nu10101498

27. Pickering, G., Mazur, A., Trousselard, M., Bienkowski, P.,
Yaltsewa, N., Amessou, M., Noah, L., & Pouteau, E. (2020).
Magnesium status and stress: The vicious circle concept revis-
ited. *Nutrients, 12*(12), 3672. https://doi.org/10.3390
/nu12123672

28. Mordarski, B. (2023). Nutrition-focused physical exam pocket
guide (3rd ed.). Academy of Nutrition and Dietetics.

29. Hrubša, M., Siatka, T., Nejmanová, I., Vopršalová, M., Kujo-
vská Krčmová, L., Matoušová, K., Javorská, L., Macáková, K.,
Mercolini, L., Remião, F., Máťuš, M., Mladěnka, P., & On Behalf
of the oemonom (2022). Biological properties of vitamins of

the B-complex, part 1: Vitamins B1, B2, B3, and B5. *Nutrients, 14*(3), 484. https://doi.org/10.3390/nu14030484

30. Jacobs, D. R., Jr., Gross, M. D., & Tapsell, L. C. (2009). Food synergy: An operational concept for understanding nutrition. *The American Journal of Clinical Nutrition, 89*(5), 1543S–1548S. https://doi.org/10.3945/ajcn.2009.26736B

31. Sahu, P., Thippeswamy, H., & Chaturvedi, S. K. (2022). Neuropsychiatric manifestations in vitamin B12 deficiency. *Vitamins and Hormones, 119*, 457–470. https://doi.org/10.1016/bs.vh.2022.01.001

32. Mordarski, B. (2023). *Nutrition-focused physical exam pocket guide* (3rd ed.). Academy of Nutrition and Dietetics.

33. Liwinsky, T., & Lang, U. E. (2023). Folate and its significance in depressive disorders and suicidality: A comprehensive narrative review. *Nutrients, 15*(17), 3859. https://doi.org/10.3390/nu15173859

34. Mordarski, B. (2023). *Nutrition-focused physical exam pocket guide* (3rd ed.). Academy of Nutrition and Dietetics.

35. Parra, M., Stahl, S., & Hellmann, H. (2018). Vitamin B_6 and its role in cell metabolism and physiology. *Cells, 7*(7), 84. https://doi.org/10.3390/cells7070084

36. Mordarski, B. (2023). *Nutrition-focused physical exam pocket guide* (3rd ed.). Academy of Nutrition and Dietetics.

37. Mordarski, B. (2023). *Nutrition-focused physical exam pocket guide* (3rd ed.). Academy of Nutrition and Dietetics.

38. Mordarski, B. (2023). *Nutrition-focused physical exam pocket guide* (3rd ed.). Academy of Nutrition and Dietetics.

Chapter 6

1. Sun, Y., Qu, Y., & Zhu, J. (2021). The relationship between
    inflammation and post-traumatic stress disorder. *Frontiers in
    Psychiatry, 12,* 707543. https://doi.org/10.3389/fpsyt.2021
    .707543

2. Olivieri, P., Solitar, B., & Dubois, M. (2012). Childhood risk fac-
    tors for developing fibromyalgia. *Open Access Rheumatology:
    Research and Reviews, 4,* 109–114. https://doi.org/10.2147
    /OARRR.S36086

3. Thurston, R. C., Chang, Y., Matthews, K. A., von Känel, R., &
    Koenen, K. (2019). Association of sexual harassment and sexual
    assault with midlife women's mental and physical health. *JAMA
    Internal Medicine, 179*(1), 48–53. https://doi.org/10.1001
    /jamainternmed.2018.4886

4. Paradies, Y., Ben, J., Denson, N., Elias, A., Priest, N., Pieterse,
    A., Gupta, A., Kelaher, M., & Gee, G. (2015). Racism as a deter-
    minant of health: A systematic review and meta-analysis. *PloS
    one, 10*(9), e0138511. https://doi.org/10.1371/journal
    .pone.0138511

5. Halpern, L. R., Shealer, M. L., Cho, R., McMichael, E. B.,
    Rogers, J., Ferguson-Young, D., Mouton, C. P., Tabatabai, M.,
    Southerland, J., & Gangula, P. (2017). Influence of intimate
    partner violence (IPV) exposure on cardiovascular and salivary
    biosensors: Is there a relationship? *Journal of the National
    Medical Association, 109*(4), 252–261. https://doi.org/10.1016
    /j.jnma.2017.08.001

6. Kiecolt-Glaser, J. K., Gouin, J. P., & Hantsoo, L. (2010). Close
    relationships, inflammation, and health. *Neuroscience and*

Biobehavioral Reviews, 35(1), 33–38. https://doi.org/10.1016/j
.neubiorev.2009.09.003

7. Kanki, M., Nath, A. P., Xiang, R., Yiallourou, S., Fuller, P. J.,
Cole, T. J., Cánovas, R., & Young, M. J. (2023). Poor sleep and
shift work associate with increased blood pressure and inflammation in UK Biobank participants. *Nature Communications,
14(*1), 7096. https://doi.org/10.1038/s41467-023-42758-6

8. Walker, W. H., 2nd, Walton, J. C., DeVries, A. C., & Nelson, R. J.
(2020). Circadian rhythm disruption and mental health. *Translational Psychiatry, 10*(1), 28. https://doi.org/10.1038/s41398
-020-0694-0

9. Voigt, R. M., Forsyth, C. B., Green, S. J., Engen, P. A., & Keshavarzian, A. (2016). Circadian rhythm and the gut microbiome.
International Review of Neurobiology, 131, 193–205. https:/
/doi.org/10.1016/bs.irn.2016.07.002

10. Guo, Z., Tan, Y., Lin, C., Li, H., Xie, Q., Lai, Z., Liang, X., Tan,
L., & Jing, C. (2025). Unraveling the connection between
endocrine-disrupting chemicals and anxiety: An integrative ep-
idemiological and bioinformatic perspective. *Ecotoxicology and
Environmental Safety, 296,* 118188. https://doi.org/10.1016/j
.ecoenv.2025.118188

11. Nersesian, P. V., Han, H. R., Yenokyan, G., Blumenthal, R. S.,
Nolan, M. T., Hladek, M. D., & Szanton, S. L. (2018). Loneli-
ness in middle age and biomarkers of systemic inflammation:
Findings from midlife in the United States. *Social Science &
Medicine (1982), 209,* 174–181. https://doi.org/10.1016/j
.socscimed.2018.04.007

12. Moieni, M., Irwin, M. R., Jevtic, I., Breen, E. C., Cho, H. J., Arevalo, J. M., Ma, J., Cole, S. W., & Eisenberger, N. I. (2015). Trait sensitivity to social disconnection enhances pro-inflammatory responses to a randomized controlled trial of endotoxin. *Psychoneuroendocrinology, 62,* 336–342. https://doi.org/10.1016/j.psyneuen.2015.08.020

Chapter 7

1. Nerurkar, A., Bitton, A., Davis, R. B., Phillips, R. S., & Yeh, G. (2013). When physicians counsel about stress: Results of a national study. *JAMA Internal Medicine, 173*(1), 76–77. https://doi.org/10.1001/2013.jamainternmed.480

2. Avey, H., Matheny, K. B., Robbins, A., & Jacobson, T. A. (2003). Health care providers' training, perceptions, and practices regarding stress and health outcomes. *Journal of the National Medical Association, 95*(9), 833–845.

3. Dana, D. A. (2021). *Anchored: How to befriend your nervous system using polyvagal theory.* Sounds True.

4. Ogle, C. M., Rubin, D. C., & Siegler, I. C. (2015). The relation between insecure attachment and posttraumatic stress: Early life versus adulthood traumas. *Psychological trauma: Theory, Research, Practice and Policy, 7*(4), 324–332. https://doi.org/10.1037/tra0000015

5. Dana, D. A. (2018). *The polyvagal theory in therapy: Engaging the rhythm of regulation.* W. W. Norton & Company.

6. Yang, Y. C., Schorpp, K., & Harris, K. M. (2014). Social support, social strain and inflammation: Evidence from a

national longitudinal study of U.S. adults. *Social Science & Medicine (1982), 107,* 124–135. https://doi.org/10.1016/j.socscimed.2014.02.013

7. Cole, S. W., Levine, M. E., Arevalo, J. M., Ma, J., Weir, D. R., & Crimmins, E. M. (2015). Loneliness, eudaimonia, and the human conserved transcriptional response to adversity. *Psycho-neuroendocrinology, 62,* 11–17. https://doi.org/10.1016/j.psyneuen.2015.07.001

8. Gee, N. R., Rodriguez, K. E., Fine, A. H., & Trammell, J. P. (2021). Dogs supporting human health and well-being: A biopsychosocial approach. *Frontiers in Veterinary Science, 8,* 630465. https://doi.org/10.3389/fvets.2021.630465

9. Saarenpää, M., Roslund, M. I., Nurminen, N., Puhakka, R., Kummola, L., Laitinen, O. H., Hyöty, H., & Sinkkonen, A. (2024). Urban indoor gardening enhances immune regulation and diversifies skin microbiota—a placebo-controlled double-blinded intervention study. *Environment International, 187,* 108705. https://doi.org/10.1016/j.envint.2024.108705

10. Li Q. (2022). Effects of forest environment (Shinrin-yoku/Forest bathing) on health promotion and disease prevention—the establishment of "Forest Medicine." *Environmental Health and Preventive Medicine, 27,* 43. https://doi.org/10.1265/ehpm.22-00160

11. Coss, R., & Keller, C. (2022). Transient decreases in blood pressure and heart rate with increased subjective level of relaxation while viewing water compared with adjacent ground. *Journal of Environmental Psychology, 81.* https://doi.org/10.1016/j.jenvp.2022.101794

12. Egerer, M., Lin, B., Kingsley, J., Marsh, P., Diekmann, L., & Ossola, A. (2022). Gardening can relieve human stress and boost nature connection during the COVID-19 pandemic. *Urban Forestry & Urban Greening, 68,* 127483. https://doi .org/10.1016/j.ufug.2022.127483

13. Soga, M., Gaston, K. J., & Yamaura, Y. (2016). Gardening is beneficial for health: A meta-analysis. *Preventive Medicine Reports, 5,* 92–99. https://doi.org/10.1016/j.pmedr.2016.11.007

14. Liu, S., Zhang, X., & Zhao, C. (2025). Happiness in the sky: The effect of sunshine exposure on subjective well-being. *Biodemography and Social Biology, 70*(2), 67–81. https://doi.org/10.1080 /19485565.2025.2487977

15. Wang, J., Wei, Z., Yao, N., Li, C., & Sun, L. (2023). Association between sunlight exposure and mental health: Evidence from a special population without sunlight in work. *Risk Management and Healthcare Policy, 16,* 1049–1057. https://doi.org/10 .2147/RMHP.S420018

16. Song, I., Keller, K. B., Kim, C., & Song, C. (2023). Effects of nature sounds on the attention and physiological and psychological relaxation. *Urban Forestry & Urban Greening, 86*(1). https://doi.org/10.1016/j.ufug.2023.127987

17. Treleaven, D. A. (2018). *Trauma-sensitive mindfulness: Practices for safe and transformative healing.* W. W. Norton & Company.

18. Twal, W. O., Wahlquist, A. E., & Balasubramanian, S. (2016). Yogic breathing when compared to attention control reduces the levels of pro-inflammatory biomarkers in saliva: A pilot randomized controlled trial. *BMC Complementary and Alternative Medicine, 16,* 294. https://doi.org/10.1186/s12906-016-1286-7

19. Vierra, J., Boonla, O., & Prasertsri, P. (2022). Effects of sleep deprivation and 4-7-8 breathing control on heart rate variability, blood pressure, blood glucose, and endothelial function in healthy young adults. *Physiological Reports, 10*(13), e15389. https://doi.org/10.14814/phy2.15389

20. Balban, M. Y., Neri, E., Kogon, M. M., Weed, L., Nouriani, B., Jo, B., Holl, G., Zeitzer, J. M., Spiegel, D., & Huberman, A. D. (2023). Brief structured respiration practices enhance mood and reduce physiological arousal. *Cell Reports, Medicine, 4*(1), 100895. https://doi.org/10.1016/j.xcrm.2022.100895

21. Maniaci, G., Daino, M., Iapichino, M., Giammanco, A., Taormina, C., Bonura, G., Sardella, Z., Carolla, G., Cammareri, P., Sberna, E., Clesi, M. F., Ferraro, L., Gambino, C. M., Ciaccio, M., Rispoli, L., La Cascia, C., La Barbera, D., & Quattrone, D. (2024). Neurobiological and anti-inflammatory effects of a deep diaphragmatic breathing technique based on neofunctional psychotherapy: A pilot rct. *Stress and Health: Journal of the International Society for the Investigation of Stress*, Article e3503. Advance online publication. https://doi.org/10.1002/smi.3503

22. Finck, C., Avila, A., Jiménez-Leal, W., Botero, J. P., Shambo, D., Hernandez, S., Reinoso-Carvalho, F., & Andonova, V. (2023). A multisensory mindfulness experience: Exploring the promotion of sensory awareness as a mindfulness practice. *Frontiers in Psychology, 14,* 1230832. https://doi.org/10.3389/fpsyg.2023.1230832

23. Maher, M. J., Rego, S. A., & Asnis, G. M. (2006). Sleep disturbances in patients with post-traumatic stress disorder: Epidemiology, impact and approaches to management. *CNS Drugs,*

20(7), 567–590. https://doi.org/10.2165/00023210
-200620070-00003

24. Lancel, M., van Marle, H. J. F., Van Veen, M. M., & van Schagen, A. M. (2021). Disturbed sleep in PTSD: Thinking beyond nightmares. *Frontiers in Psychiatry, 12,* 767760. https://doi.org/10.3389/fpsyt.2021.767760

25. Engert, L.C., Besedovsky, L. Sleep and inflammation: A bidirectional relationship. *Somnologie* 29, 3–9 (2025). https://doi.org/10.1007/s11818-025-00495-6

26. Vernia, F., Di Ruscio, M., Ciccone, A., Viscido, A., Frieri, G., Stefanelli, G., & Latella, G. (2021). Sleep disorders related to nutrition and digestive diseases: A neglected clinical condition. *International Journal of Medical Sciences, 18*(3), 593–603. https://doi.org/10.7150/ijms.45512

27. Rusch, H. L., Rosario, M., Levison, L. M., Olivera, A., Livingston, W. S., Wu, T., & Gill, J. M. (2019). The effect of mindfulness meditation on sleep quality: A systematic review and meta-analysis of randomized controlled trials. *Annals of the New York Academy of Sciences, 1445*(1), 5–16. https://doi.org/10.1111/nyas.13996

28. Nakshine, V. S., Thute, P., Khatib, M. N., & Sarkar, B. (2022). Increased screen time as a cause of declining physical, psychological health, and sleep patterns: A literary review. *Cureus, 14*(10), e30051. https://doi.org/10.7759/cureus.30051

29. Riemann, D., Espie, C. A., Altena, E., Arnardottir, E. S., Baglioni, C., Bassetti, C. L. A., Bastien, C., Berzina, N., Bjorvatn, B., Dikeos, D., Dolenc Groselj, L., Ellis, J. G., Garcia-Borreguero,

D., Geoffroy, P. A., Gjerstad, M., Gonçalves, M., Hertenstein, E., Hoedlmoser, K., Hion, T., Holzinger, B., & Spiegelhalder, K. (2023). The European insomnia guideline: An update on the diagnosis and treatment of insomnia 2023. *Journal of Sleep Research, 32*(6), e14035. https://doi.org/10.1111/jsr.14035

30. Ekholm, B., Spulber, S., & Adler, M. (2020). A randomized controlled study of weighted chain blankets for insomnia in psychiatric disorders. *Journal of Clinical Sleep Medicine, 16*(9), 1567–1577. https://doi.org/10.5664/jcsm.8636

31. Zhang, Y., Ren, R., Yang, L., Zhou, J., Sanford, L. D., & Tang, X. (2019). The effect of treating obstructive sleep apnea with continuous positive airway pressure on posttraumatic stress disorder: A systematic review and meta-analysis with hypothetical model. *Neuroscience and Biobehavioral Reviews, 102,* 172–183. https://doi.org/10.1016/j.neubiorev.2019.03.019

32. Pence, P. G., Katz, L. S., Huffman, C., & Cojucar, G. (2014). Delivering integrative restoration-yoga nidra meditation (iRest®) to women with sexual trauma at a veteran's medical center: A pilot study. *International Journal of Yoga Therapy, 24,* 53–62.

33. Laukkanen, J. A., Laukkanen, T., & Kunutsor, S. K. (2018). Cardiovascular and other health benefits of sauna bathing: A review of the evidence. *Mayo Clinic Proceedings, 93*(8), 1111–1121. https://doi.org/10.1016/j.mayocp.2018.04.008

34. Li, S., Liu, J., Zhang, R., & Dong, J. (2024). Association study of depressive symptoms and periodontitis in an obese population: Analysis based on NHANES data from 2009 to 2014. *PloS One, 19*(12), e0315754. https://doi.org/10.1371/journal.pone.0315754

35. Simpson, C. A., Adler, C., du Plessis, M. R., Landau, E. R., Dashper, S. G., Reynolds, E. C., Schwartz, O. S., & Simmons, J. G. (2020). Oral microbiome composition, but not diversity, is associated with adolescent anxiety and depression symptoms. *Physiology & Behavior, 226,* 113126. https://doi.org/10.1016/j.physbeh.2020.113126

36. White, A. M., Giblin, L., & Boyd, L. D. (2017). The prevalence of dental anxiety in dental practice settings. *Journal of Dental Hygiene: JDH, 91*(1), 30–34.

37. Stubbs, B., Vancampfort, D., Rosenbaum, S., Firth, J., Cosco, T., Veronese, N., Salum, G. A., & Schuch, F. B. (2017). An examination of the anxiolytic effects of exercise for people with anxiety and stress-related disorders: A meta-analysis. *Psychiatry Research, 249,* 102–108. https://doi.org/10.1016/j.psychres.2016.12.020

38. Hall, K. S., Hoerster, K. D., & Yancy, W. S., Jr. (2015). Post-traumatic stress disorder, physical activity, and eating behaviors. *Epidemiologic Reviews, 37,* 103–115. https://doi.org/10.1093/epirev/mxu011

39. Lin, Y., Dai, R., Vogelaar, G., & Rinkevich, Y. (2024). Organ dependency on fascia connective tissue. *American Journal of Physiology. Cell physiology, 327*(2), C357–C361. https://doi.org/10.1152/ajpcell.00350.2024

40. Ribeiro, F. M., Petriz, B., Marques, G., Kamilla, L. H., & Franco, O. L. (2021). Is there an exercise-intensity threshold capable of avoiding the leaky gut? *Frontiers in Nutrition, 8,* 627289. https://doi.org/10.3389/fnut.2021.627289

41. Streeter, C. C., Gerbarg, P. L., Saper, R. B., Ciraulo, D. A., & Brown, R. P. (2012). Effects of yoga on the autonomic nervous system, gamma-aminobutyric-acid, and allostasis in epilepsy, depression, and post-traumatic stress disorder. *Medical Hypotheses, 78*(5), 571–579. https://doi.org/10.1016/j.mehy.2012.01.021

42. Xiong, G. L., & Doraiswamy, P. M. (2009). Does meditation enhance cognition and brain plasticity? *Annals of the New York Academy of Sciences, 1172,* 63–69. https://doi.org/10.1196/annals.1393.002

Chapter 8

1. Schinder, A. F., & Poo, M. (2000). The neurotrophin hypothesis for synaptic plasticity. *Trends in Neurosciences, 23*(12), 639–645. https://doi.org/10.1016/s0166-2236(00)01672-6

2. Ng, Q. X., Soh, A. Y. S., Loke, W., Venkatanarayanan, N., Lim, D. Y., & Yeo, W. S. (2019). Systematic review with meta-analysis: The association between post-traumatic stress disorder and irritable bowel syndrome. *Journal of Gastroenterology and Hepatology, 34*(1), 68–73. https://doi.org/10.1111/jgh.14446

3. Fritz, J., Coffey, R., Bloch, J., Cutler, A., Gabrielson, S., DiGiovanni, S., & Faherty, L. J. (2025). The relationship between adverse childhood experiences and disorders of the gut-brain interaction. *Journal of Pediatric Gastroenterology and Nutrition, 80*(1), 100–107. https://doi.org/10.1002/jpn3.12422

4. Paras, M. L., Murad, M. H., Chen, L. P., Goranson, E. N., Sattler, A. L., Colbenson, K. M., Elamin, M. B., Seime, R. J., Prokop, L.

J., & Zirakzadeh, A. (2009). Sexual abuse and lifetime diagnosis of somatic disorders: A systematic review and meta-analysis. *JAMA, 302*(5), 550–561. https://doi.org/10.1001/jama .2009.1091

5. Okazaki, Y., Yoshida, S., Kashima, S., Miyamori, D., & Matsumoto, M. (2022). Increased prescriptions for irritable bowel syndrome after the 2018 Japan floods: A longitudinal analysis based on the Japanese National Database of Health Insurance Claims and Specific Health Checkups. *BMC Gastroenterology, 22*(1), 263. https://doi.org/10.1186/s12876-022-02342-6

6. Nass, B. Y. S., Dibbets, P., & Markus, C. R. (2023). The impact of psychotrauma and emotional stress vulnerability on physical and mental functioning of patients with inflammatory bowel disease. *International Journal of Environmental Research and Public Health, 20*(21), 6976. https://doi.org/10.3390 /ijerph20216976

7. Lee, Y. B., Yu, J., Choi, H. H., Jeon, B. S., Kim, H. K., Kim, S. W., Kim, S. S., Park, Y. G., & Chae, H. S. (2017). The association between peptic ulcer diseases and mental health problems: A population-based study: A STROBE compliant article. *Medicine, 96*(34), e7828. https://doi.org/10.1097 /MD.0000000000007828

8. Shah, A., Lee, Y. Y., Suzuki, H., Tan-Loh, J., Siah, K. T. H., Gwee, K. A., Fairlie, T., Talley, N. J., Ghoshal, U. C., Wang, Y. P., Kim, Y. S., & Holtmann, G. (2024). A pathophysiologic framework for the overlap of disorders of gut-brain interaction and the role of the gut microbiome. *Gut Microbes, 16*(1), 2413367. https:/ /doi.org/10.1080/19490976.2024.2413367

9. Warren, A., Nyavor, Y., Beguelin, A., & Frame, L. A. (2024).

Dangers of the chronic stress response in the context of the microbiota-gut-immune-brain axis and mental health: A narrative review. *Frontiers in Immunology, 15,* 1365871. https://doi .org/10.3389/fimmu.2024.1365871

10. Peters, S. L., Muir, J. G., & Gibson, P. R. (2015). Review article: Gut-directed hypnotherapy in the management of irritable bowel syndrome and inflammatory bowel disease. *Alimentary Pharmacology & Therapeutics, 41*(11), 1104–1115. https://doi .org/10.1111/apt.13202

11. Pemberton, L., Kita, L., & Andrews, K. (2020). Practitioners' experiences of using Gut Directed Hypnosis for irritable bowel syndrome: Perceived impact upon client wellbeing: A qualitative study. *Complementary Therapies in Medicine, 55,* 102605. https://doi.org/10.1016/j.ctim.2020.102605

12. Jacobson, E. Spastic esophagus and mucous colitis: etiology and treatment by progressive relaxation. *Arch Intern Med, 1927,* 39, 433–445.

13. Palsson, O. S. (2006). Standardized hypnosis treatment for irritable bowel syndrome: The North Carolina protocol. *The International Journal of Clinical and Experimental Hypnosis, 54*(1), 51–64. https://doi.org/10.1080/00207140500322933

14. Palsson, O. S., & van Tilburg, M. (2015). Hypnosis and guided imagery treatment for gastrointestinal disorders: Experience with scripted Protocols developed at the University of North Carolina. *The American Journal of Clinical Hypnosis, 58*(1), 5–21. https://doi.org/10.1080/00029157.2015 .1012705

15. Whorwell, P. J., Prior, A., & Faragher, E. B. (1984). Controlled trial of hypnotherapy in the treatment of severe refractory irritable-bowel syndrome. *Lancet (London, England), 2*(8414), 1232–1234. https://doi.org/10.1016/s0140-6736(84)92793-4

16. Peter, J., Fournier, C., Keip, B., Rittershaus, N., Stephanou-Rieser, N., Durdevic, M., Dejaco, C., Michalski, M., & Moser, G. (2018). Intestinal microbiome in irritable bowel syndrome before and after gut-directed hypnotherapy. *International Journal of Molecular Sciences, 19*(11), 3619. https://doi.org/10.3390/ijms19113619

Chapter 9

1. Voigt, R. M., Forsyth, C. B., Green, S. J., Engen, P. A., & Keshavarzian, A. (2016). Circadian rhythm and the gut microbiome. *International Review of Neurobiology, 131,* 193–205. https://doi.org/10.1016/bs.irn.2016.07.002

2. Rathore, K., Shukla, N., Naik, S., Sambhav, K., Dange, K., Bhuyan, D., & Imranul Haq, Q. M. (2025). The bidirectional relationship between the gut microbiome and mental health: A comprehensive review. *Cureus, 17*(3), e80810. https://doi.org/10.7759/cureus.80810

3. Decandia, D., Gelfo, F., Landolfo, E., Balsamo, F., Petrosini, L., & Cutuli, D. (2023). Dietary protection against cognitive impairment, neuroinflammation and oxidative stress in alzheimer's disease animal models of lipopolysaccharide-induced inflammation. *International Journal of Molecular Sciences, 24*(6), 5921. https://doi.org/10.3390/ijms24065921

4. Liu, L., Zhang, Q., Cai, Y., Sun, D., He, X., Wang, L., Yu, D., Li, X., Xiong, X., Xu, H., Yang, Q., & Fan, X. (2016). Resveratrol counteracts lipopolysaccharide-induced depressive-like behaviors via enhanced hippocampal neurogenesis. *Oncotarget, 7*(35), 56045–56059. https://doi.org/10.18632/oncotarget.11178

5. Xiao, Y., Yang, C., Si, N., Chu, T., Yu, J., Yuan, X., & Chen, X. T. (2024). Epigallocatechin-3-gallate inhibits LPS/AβO-induced neuroinflammation in BV2 cells through regulating the ROS/TXNIP/NLRP3 pathway. *Journal of Neuroimmune Pharmacology, 19*(1), 31. https://doi.org/10.1007/s11481-024-10131-z

6. Decandia, D., Gelfo, F., Landolfo, E., Balsamo, F., Petrosini, L., & Cutuli, D. (2023). Dietary protection against cognitive impairment, neuroinflammation and oxidative stress in alzheimer's disease animal models of lipopolysaccharide-induced inflammation. *International Journal of Molecular Sciences, 24*(6), 5921. https://doi.org/10.3390/ijms24065921

7. Jin, L., Wu, L., Zhu, G., Yang, L., Zhao, D., He, J., & Zhang, Y. (2025). Association between dietary flavonoid intake and anxiety: Data from NHANES 2017-2018. *BMC Public Health, 25*(1), 1477. https://doi.org/10.1186/s12889-025-22621-7

8. Magnúsdóttir, S., Ravcheev, D., de Crécy-Lagard, V., & Thiele, I. (2015). Systematic genome assessment of B-vitamin biosynthesis suggests co-operation among gut microbes. *Frontiers in Genetics, 6,* 148. https://doi.org/10.3389/fgene.2015.00148

9. Satoh, K., Hazama, M., Maeda-Yamamoto, M., & Nishihira, J. (2025). Relationship between dietary habits and stress responses exerted by different gut microbiota. *Nutrients, 17*(8), 1388. https://doi.org/10.3390/nu17081388

10. Brenner, L. A., Stearns-Yoder, K. A., Stamper, C. E., Hoisington, A. J., Brostow, D. P., Hoffmire, C. A., Forster, J. E., Donovan, M. L., Ryan, A. T., Postolache, T. T., & Lowry, C. A. (2022). Rationale, design, and methods: A randomized placebo-controlled trial of an immunomodulatory probiotic intervention for veterans with PTSD. *Contemporary Clinical Trials Communications, 28,* 100960. https://doi.org/10.1016/j.conctc.2022.100960

11. Savignac, H. M., Kiely, B., Dinan, T. G., & Cryan, J. F. (2014). Bifidobacteria exert strain-specific effects on stress-related behavior and physiology in BALB/c mice. *Neurogastroenterology and Motility, 26*(11), 1615–1627. https://doi.org/10.1111/nmo.12427

12. Messaoudi, M., Violle, N., Bisson, J. F., Desor, D., Javelot, H., & Rougeot, C. (2011). Beneficial psychological effects of a probiotic formulation (Lactobacillus helveticus R0052 and Bifidobacterium longum R0175) in healthy human volunteers. *Gut Microbes, 2*(4), 256–261. https://doi.org/10.4161/gmic.2.4.16108

13. Kato-Kataoka, A., Nishida, K., Takada, M., Kawai, M., Kikuchi-Hayakawa, H., Suda, K., Ishikawa, H., Gondo, Y., Shimizu, K., Matsuki, T., Kushiro, A., Hoshi, R., Watanabe, O., Igarashi, T., Miyazaki, K., Kuwano, Y., & Rokutan, K. (2016). Fermented milk containing lactobacillus casei strain Shirota preserves the diversity of the gut microbiota and relieves abdominal dysfunction in healthy medical students exposed to academic stress. *Applied and Environmental Microbiology, 82*(12), 3649–3658. https://doi.org/10.1128/AEM.04134-15

14. Steenbergen, L., Sellaro, R., van Hemert, S., Bosch, J. A., & Colzato, L. S. (2015). A randomized controlled trial to test the effect of multispecies probiotics on cognitive reactivity to sad mood. *Brain, Behavior, and Immunity, 48,* 258–264. https://doi.org/10.1016/j.bbi.2015.04.003

Chapter 10

1. [Sounds True Insights at the Edge]. (2020, June 16). *Befriending your nervous system* [Video]. Sounds True. https://resources.soundstrue.com/transcript/deb-dana-befriending-your-nervous-system/

2. Wu, J., Pierart, C., Chaplin, T. M., Hommer, R. E., Mayes, L. C., & Crowley, M. J. (2020). Getting to the heart of food craving with resting heart rate variability in adolescents. *Appetite, 155,* 104816. https://doi.org/10.1016/j.appet.2020.104816

3. Godfrey, K. M., Juarascio, A., Manasse, S., Minassian, A., Risbrough, V., & Afari, N. (2019). Heart rate variability and emotion regulation among individuals with obesity and loss of control eating. *Physiology & Behavior, 199,* 73–78. https://doi.org/10.1016/j.physbeh.2018.11.009

4. Karemaker, J. M. (2022). The multibranched nerve: Vagal function beyond heart rate variability. *Biological Psychology, 172,* 108378. https://doi.org/10.1016/j.biopsycho.2022.108378

About the Author

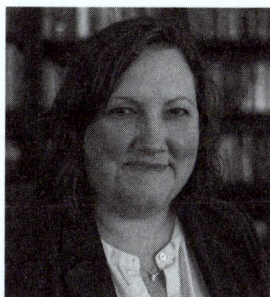

Meg Bowman is a licensed nutritionist, educator, and author who specializes in the intersection of mental health and nutrition. She is the cofounder of several organizations that reflect her commitment to functional, compassionate, and evidence-based care.

She cofounded Nutrition Hive (www.nutritionhive.health), a functional group nutrition practice where she works with clients navigating mental health and gastrointestinal conditions.

At Clinician's Incubator (www.cliniciansincubator.com), Meg mentors postgraduate nutrition professionals pursuing the Certified Nutrition Specialist (CNS) credential, offering clinical supervision, test preparation, and business development support.

She is also cofounder and a faculty member at Nested Health Coach Certification (www.nestedhealthcoach.com), an NBHWC-approved certification program designed specifically for providers.

The program integrates trauma-informed approaches, polyvagal theory, and coaching tools for working with clients navigating complex health challenges.

You can learn more about Meg and her work at
www.megbowmannutrition.com.